Tri

The New Self Treatment Guide to Pain Relief

Dr. Michelle Ellen Gleen

Free Bonus

Download my **"Keto Cookbook with 60+ Keto Recipes For Your Personal Enjoyment"** Ebook For **FREE!**

The **Keto Diet Cookbook** is a collection of **60+ delicious recipes** that are easy and fun to make in the comfort of your own home. It gives you the exact *recipes that you can use to prepare meals for any moment of the day, breakfast, lunch, dinner, and even dessert.*

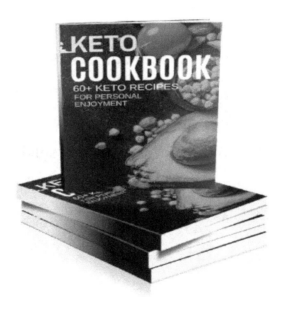

You don't need 5 different cookbooks with a ton of recipes to live a healthy and fun lifestyle. *You just need a good and efficient one and that is what the **Keto Diet Cookbook** is.*

Click the URL below to Download the Book For FREE, and also Subscribe for Free books, giveaways, and new releases by me. https://mayobook.com/drmichelle

My Books

Alkaline Diet: The Secret to Healthy Living with Alkaline Foods (Healthy Food Lifestyle)

The Alkaline Diet Cookbook: Your Guide to Eating More Alkaline Foods, and Less Acidic Foods For Healthy Living (Healthy Food Lifestyle)

Ketogenic Diet For Beginners: Your Complete Keto Guide and Cookbook with Low Carb, High-Fat Recipes For Living The Keto Lifestyle

Anti Inflammatory Diet Cookbook For Beginners: 3-Week Quick & Delicious Meal Plan with Easy Recipes to Heal The Immune Systems and Restore Overall Health

Apple Cider Vinegar: A Quick, Easy, and Affordable Guide to the Health Benefits, and Healing Power of Apple Cider Vinegar (ACV)

Apple Cider Vinegar: The Amazing Guide on The Uses of ACV For Numerous Health Conditions, and How to Make it from Home

Brain Cancer Awareness: How to Help Your Brain Fight Brain Cancer

Dr. Sebi Cookbook: Alkaline Diet Nutritional Guide with Sea moss, Medicinal Herbal Teas, Smoothies, Desserts, Mushroom, Salads, Soups & More, to Rejuvenate the Body with 100+ Recipes

Skin Tag Removal: How To Get Rid of Your Skin Tags in Simple

Steps

Trigger Points: The New Self Treatment Guide to Pain Relief

Table of Contents

Introduction

How would you like to be able to reduce pain without ever taking pills?

Trigger Points is a guide to help people identify, understand, and manage pain and discomfort. The ultimate goal of Trigger Points is to make you feel better. But the first step is understanding how your body works, and figuring out which treatment methods will work best for you. Trigger Points is a revolutionary new self treatment guide to pain relief.

This book is not intended to diagnose, treat or cure any medical conditions; rather, it will help you get started on the path to healing yourself by using an effective self-treatment guide for pain relief.

Trigger points are a group of muscles that become stuck in a painful position and are often referred to as "knots" or "tender points".

This book is a self-help guide to using trigger points and deep tissue massage as a safe and effective alternative to traditional treatments for pain relief. While massage can be helpful, many people find that it's hard to make a commitment to treatment. They'd rather just treat themselves at home or at work with the tools they already have in their cabinets. The best part about trigger points and deep tissue massage is that it's safe, cheap and effective. All you need is a basic set of supplies, some patience and a willingness to learn.

We all know the importance of exercise, but let's face it, most of us only know how to do a few simple things. Most of us don't have a proper understanding of anatomy and physiology, and we haven't been taught how to exercise properly. If you're like most people, you probably only understand half of the body's trigger points, and you probably have no idea how to prevent them.

"Trigger points" are tender spots that form when a muscle is repeatedly overused. They are located between the muscles and tendons, but only touch the skin. The main purpose of trigger points is to provide relief from pain, not treat it. They are caused by chronic muscle strain or poor posture. Trigger points are a sign of tension and stress and need to be addressed to relieve the pain. The best way to reduce trigger points is to work on the entire body. Strengthening the muscles will strengthen the nerves and relieve pain. The muscles also relax

naturally with time, which helps prevent the formation of trigger points. Some exercises to relieve trigger points are as follows:

- Sit in a chair with your back straight and your feet flat on the floor. Keep your spine relaxed. Your knees should be slightly bent. Your elbows should be resting on the armrests.

- Exhale and press down gently with your hands to lower your upper back onto the chair. You can use your arms to help you lower your back. You can also push your hips backward while pressing your palms down. When you have lowered your back to the height that feels comfortable, hold this position for five to 10 seconds.

- Inhale and slowly lift your head and shoulders up to the original position.

- Repeat this exercise five to ten times.

Trigger points (also known as *myofascial trigger points*) are painful knots or fibrous structures that develop in muscle tissue and fascia. *Myofascial trigger points* are frequently seen in the neck, shoulders, back, hip girdle, and knee. The pain associated with these trigger points is caused by the local contractions of muscles, which are usually brought about by the stretching of tendons and ligaments.

In addition, the sensation of pain in the affected area can be felt deep in the muscle tissue.

You've tried everything—from acupuncture to prescription pain medication, but nothing seems to work. And if you're like most people, you've tried everything from heat packs to chiropractic adjustments. *"Trigger Points: The New Self Treatment Guide to Pain Relief"* is the definitive book on trigger point therapy, the most effective and natural form of massage available.

One of the best areas of muscle mass for inducing pain is the inducer/trigger point. A result in a position at the back, for example, may produce a recommendation pain in the throat. As a satellite, the throat brings about the end and subsequent distress at the top. The discomfort can range from a sharp stabbing pain to a dull ache.

The purpose of trigger point therapeutic massage is to relieve pain at its source by applying and releasing pressure in isolated areas. Yoga breathing and determining the precise location and intensity of pain are both part of this type of trigger point therapy massage therapy.

Trigger point massage results in the release of constrictions in the muscles, resulting in pain relief. After only one treatment, you may notice a significant reduction in pain. Frequent therapeutic massage with active point therapy can help alleviate chronic pain and anxiety.

An **induce point** *(also known as a "trigger point")* is a painful nodule located in the fascia of the skeletal muscles that is particularly sensitive. Muscle contractions and direct compression can result in a leap indication, local tenderness, local twitch response, and known pain that can be felt miles away.

It is a characteristic of behavior to respond to pressure on the trigger point that jumps out. Extreme pain frequently shocks people. Depending on their reaction, they may wince or even weep, which is strange considering the amount of pressure applied by the analyzing fingertips. They jerk the glenohumeral joint, the head, or other parts of the body that cannot be palpated involuntarily. *The trigger point's* excessive soreness is reflected in a jump indication. Pathognomonic for the presence of ***trigger points***, this sign has long been taken as a sign of disease.

Local twitch response: Nervous muscle fibers twitch when pressure is applied to them, resulting in a temporary visible or palpable contraction of the muscles and skin. This can be brought on by needle penetration or transverse snapping.

When a person feels pain in a location other than where they were hit by the painful stimulus, this is referred to as **"reflective pain."** No matter where the source of the pain is located, it can be reliably reproduced. In this case, there is no evidence of joint inflammation or neurological impairment. Having a myofascial trigger point means that you have a specific, discrete, and continuous pattern of pain that doesn't change based on race or gender and that can be repeated.

A myocardial infarction may cause a patient to experience radiating pain in the upper body, or it may be referred pain that is known. When a person only has pain in their jaw or remaining arm, but not in the upper body, they are experiencing referred pain, which is the opposite of direct pain.

Chapter 1

Anatomy and Etiology

It is in the myofascial area where the engine endplate penetrates that trigger factors are formed *(main or central trigger points)*. Pliable nodules in the muscle as large as 2–10 mm can be felt in almost any skeletal muscle of the body. Trigger points are found in nearly everyone's torso. Even in children and newborns, it can be present, but this does not always lead to the development of pain symptoms. In the case of trigger points, symptoms of myofascial pain, physical dysfunction, mental disturbance, and restricted daily work are all directly linked to them.

Those who suffer from the *Myofascial Pain Syndrome* experience muscle tenderness and localized pain in their muscles and fascia caused by tiny, painful trigger points, also known as trigger points, which have a diameter of only a few millimeters.

The common causes of trigger points are Due to:

- Aging.

- Falling, tension, or delivery trauma might cause injury.

- Insufficient exercise: Men make up 45 percent of all sedentary people between the ages of 27 and 55.

- Strength training, weightlifting, and sitting cross-legged are all examples of activities that can lead to poor posture.

- Emotional stress and trauma can cause a long-term state of anxiety or depression.

- Insufficient intake of vitamins C, D, B, folate, and iron; sleep disturbances; joint pain and hypermobility; and inadequate intake of vitamins C, D, and B.

Identifying and Classifying Trigger Points

There are two types of trigger points: Main (or central) and Supplementary (or satellite).

According to a referred-pain map, *Main or central trigger sites* are the ones that generate the most severe pain when applied to the area of the body. The intestines of the muscle bellies tend to be the focus of these exercises.

Trigger points in surrounding muscles can cause *Supplementary or satellite trigger points* to form. It's very common for trigger point healing to make the cluster dissipate, but it could still be there in a well-executed grouping of trigger points.

Active and inactive Trigger points

Tenderness and a referred pain pattern are signs of an **active trigger point**. Trigger points in the center, as well as a few outlying trigger points, are more frequently active (although not necessarily most of them). Provoking factors can lead to the activation of previously inactive trigger sites.

When a **trigger point is inactive**, it feels like a mass under the fingertips. They can cause the muscles to become more tense.

Diffuse Trigger Points

When there is a severe postural deformity, it is common for there to be many primary trigger points, leading to the emergence of secondary, or "*diffuse*," trigger points.

Attachment Activate Points

Arise at the very delicate tendon-osseous connections. A nearby joint may begin to degenerate if it is not addressed.

Ligamentous Induce Points

There are trigger sites in the ligaments as well. It's possible to develop throat instability if there are trigger points in the anterior longitudinal ligament of the backbone. Leg pain disorders such as ligament patellae and fibular security ligament, for example, can be successfully treated.

Theories of Pathogenesis

The formation of trigger points remains a mystery. The emergence, sensitization, and manifestation of trigger points have been the subject of several theories, but only a few have been supported by empirical evidence.

Thin Myelinated and unmyelinated fibers are involved in transmitting pain from trigger points in normal circumstances. If you think about it, trigger points are probably caused by the activation and sensitization of the A and C fibers by a variety of painful and non-painful things, such as mechanical stimuli or chemical agents.

Today's working hypothesis is the ITPH *(Integrated Result in Point Hypothesis)*. Multiple factors can cause sarcomere overactivation, which results in pathogenic alterations at the molecular level. Endogenous (involuntary) shortening of muscle fibers and an increase in metabolic load on local cells occur as a result of this becoming totally sarcomeres. According to electrophysiological studies, the electrical activity at trigger points is caused by malfunctioning extra-fuse engine endplates, not by muscle spindles as previously thought.

- **The polymodal theory** describes the presence of polymodal receptors (PMRs) throughout your body, which become induced sites in the presence of certain continuous, pathogenic inputs.

- In **radiculopathy theory**, problems with nerve roots are directly linked to neurovascular markers in the immediate vicinity and far away.

- **Central and Peripheral Sensitization**: In addition to peripheral sensitization, central sensitization is becoming more common, which can help explain chronic or severe pain. A reversible increase in excitability and synaptic potency of neurons in the primary nociceptive pathway is unmistakably caused by central sensitization in response to severe or recurrent stimulation of the nociceptor in the periphery. Hypersensitivity to pain is one of the symptoms *(called tactile allodynia and hyperalgesia supplementary to puncture or pressure)*. Electrophysiological or imaging techniques may be used to detect these alterations in the central nervous system.

Differential Diagnosis

Fibromyalgia is perceived as scattered tiredness and aches all across the body. Women are more likely than males to have sensitive areas in their muscles, bones, tendons, ligaments, and body fat, which are more common in women than in men. Tenderness over soft cells causes local pain and is palpable, although patients do not show leap signs when pressed or known pain maps when soft components are present. A full examination by an experienced physician is necessary to distinguish between these two pain syndromes, although they may be concurrent and connected.

Muscle pain, for example, can lead to:

- Musculoskeletal diseases
- Occupational myalgias.
- Post-traumatic hyperirritability syndrome.
- Joint dysfunction (osteoarthritis).
- Tendonitis and bursitis.
- Neurological disorders.
- Trigeminal neuralgia.
- Glossopharyngeal neuralgia.
- Sphenopalatine neuralgia
- Systemic diseases
- The systemic lupus erythematosus (SLE).
- Rheumatoid arthritis.
- Gout.
- Psoriatic arthritis.

- Infections (viral, bacterial, protozoan, parasitic and Candidiasis infection)

- Lyme disease

- Hypoglycemia and Hypothyroidism.

- Heterotopic pain of central origin.

- Axis II-type disorders.

- Psychogenic pain.

- Intensely distressing actions

Diagnoses and Observations

Chronic pain disorders (*ex-lover: headaches, pains all over, stiffness in the morning, TMJ symptoms, tinnitus, etc.*) are the most common reason why someone seeks care, and they are oftentimes the source of that suffering.

Modifications to Adaptability (ROM)

Exacerbating symptoms by making you move in an uncomfortable way or do something you dislike. Symptoms include tension headaches, migraines, ringing in the ears, and TMJ issues. In addition, there are irregularities in posture and compensatory movements.

Diagnostic Procedures

Trigger points can't be diagnosed using a lab test or imaging technique.

Anamnesis: A patient's recollection of their medical history should be detailed. It is imperative that the individual be questioned about fibromyalgia as well as whether or not it is present in their family's medical history. It's also a good idea to inquire about the patient's daily activities and physical activity, as they may be considered risk factors for depression. How long have you used your muscles? How much stress do you put yourself under each day? Do you take drugs? Do you have problems sleeping? In addition, questions about (chronic) muscle overuse, daily stress, drugs (and their overuse), and sleep disturbances must be thoroughly investigated.

Examination

To begin, feel for the exact spot and trigger point. Look for nodules or lumps in the muscles or fascia (little or large), as well as a change in temperature in the area of active trigger points (pores and skin warmer or more relaxed). Other signs to look out for include:

- The start of discomfort and the recurrence of pain are both muscular in nature.

- At the site of the trigger point discomfort, there is reproducible muscular tenderness.

- When the trigger point is mechanically activated, pain can be referred locally or far away from the site of the trigger point soreness. This muscle-specific pain and tenderness mimics the location of the patient's complaint.

A tight band of muscle fibers running across the painful area of a shortened muscle is always visible as a palpable hardening *(just like a string on a guitar)*.

When the activation point is stimulated, a twitching response occurs in the taut flesh.

Palpation can be done standing, seated, or prone, depending on the patient's preference. The ROM test and a postural assessment are also required.

Indicators of the End Result

When it comes to documenting trigger points, Fischer suggests using an algometer (*pressure threshold meter*). This meter may also be used to measure physical therapy outcomes. A greater number of results were found for pressure pain threshold and visual analogue level (VAS) ratings in the tests that were examined. ROM can also be used as a tool for evaluating therapy.

Medical Management

Medications: For mild discomfort, Tylenol (*acetaminophen*) and non-steroidal anti-inflammatory drugs (NSAIDs) such as aspirin, ibuprofen, and naproxen can be used to treat mild discomfort. Both acetaminophen and nonsteroidal anti-inflammatory drugs (NSAIDs) relieve pain and edema caused by muscle aches and stiffness (*inflammation and discomfort*). If over-the-counter medications do not offer any relief (*Vicodin*), anti-anxiety meds (*Valium*), antidepressants (*Cymbalta*), NSAIDs such as Celebrex, or a brief course of more potent painkillers (*codeine*), hydrocodone, and acetaminophen may be prescribed if over-the-counter medications do not offer any relief (*Vicodin*).

When a needle is inserted into the patient's active trigger point (ATP), the procedure is known as "***Point Injection***" (TPI). Corticosteroids can be added to the anesthetic or saline injection. The trigger point is rendered dormant and the associated discomfort is reduced thanks to the infusion. Long-lasting relief can often be achieved with only a few sessions of treatment. Shots are administered by your doctor and normally last only for a brief period of time. Injections can be administered to a number of different locations at the same time. A dry-needle approach (in which no medications are used) can be utilized if a patient has an allergic response to a certain medication.

Physical Therapy Management

- There should be a focus on reducing or eliminating trigger points in daily life whenever possible, as well as on posture and lifestyle training and education.

- There are three types of exercises that can be done daily: passive stretching, foam roller extending, and deep-stroke therapeutic massage.

- **Strengthening**: There is a progression from simple isometrics to isotonics.

- Trigger point ischemia is created in the trigger point zone with the use of continuous pressure, which has been referred to as an **Ischemic Compression Technique**. However, the trigger point's nucleus is hypoxic, which makes this theory doubtful. Despite this, Simons detailed the same therapeutic method, with no need for further ischemia in the trigger point area (Trigger Point Pressure Release). Sarcomeres within the trigger point are to be freed by this system. A small amount of pressure is all that is needed to ease the tension in the trigger point area without causing any discomfort. After therapy, the range of motion (ROM) improves significantly in both procedures.

Taping Technique

Due to trigger points, manual lymphatic drainage (MLD) should be used in conjunction with ethyl chloride spray and extended technique.

Reciprocal Inhibition (RI), Post-Isometric Relaxation (PIR), Contract-Relax/Hold-Relax (CRHR), Contract-Relax/Antagonist Contract (CR/AC) are other neuromuscular strategies (CRAC).

There are a number of particular methods, including Neuromuscular Technique, Myotherapy (MT), Ultrasound, Diathermy-Tecar Therapy, Laser Beam, and Ionophoresis.

Other managements

There are a variety of treatments that have been documented in books.

Please note that not every one of these topics is supported by substantial scientific evidence. It's possible that immediate benefits following treatment could occur due to placebo-effects in most trials because they aren't all placebo-controlled.

Laser therapy, Prolotherapy, and Dry Needling are some of the treatments available (injecting solutions around trigger points: lidocaine, glycerine, phenol).

Chapter 2

Benefits of Induce Point Therapy

As an optional treatment, inducing points can be beneficial in identifying and releasing results at specific points. When compressed, these sites cause pain in the skeletal muscle. Trigger points frequently occur as a result of muscle fiber damage.

Trigger point therapy, also known as ***myofascial trigger point therapy or neuromuscular therapy***, is most commonly used to treat pain-related problems. Therapeutic massage, chiropractic care, and dry-out needling can all be used to get rid of trigger points.

Induced Point Therapy: Its Many Uses

Trigger point therapy is used in alternative medicine to treat a wide range of chronic pain disorders, including: headaches, temporomandibular joint discomfort, and low back pain.

As a result, trigger point treatment is used to treat osteoarthritis, carpal tunnel syndrome and symptoms, tinnitus, migraines, sciatica, and sports injuries.

Traditional Acupuncture vs. Induced Point Therapy

Dry needling is a frequent method of trigger point therapy that involves putting a needle *(without the use of medicine or injection)* into the source of the problem. If you confuse dry needling with acupuncture, which uses needles to stimulate variables considered to relate to routes that bring vital energy (or *"chi"*) throughout the body, you're missing out on a lot of benefits.

Trigger point therapy is not focused on improving the flow of chi because there are some overlaps between trigger point sites and acupuncture points. Acupuncture can be used to treat a wide range of health issues, but active point therapy is predominantly utilized to address musculoskeletal diseases.

Back Pain

As a complementary therapy, dry needling may be useful for people with chronic lower back pain. According to a 2005 Cochrane Data source of Organized Reviews review, such is the conclusion. Nevertheless, due to the large number of low-quality papers evaluated, the authors of the study remind us that additional research is required on the effectiveness of dried out needling in treating low back pain.

Headaches

A 2012 paper from Expert Overview of Neurotherapeutics found that trigger point therapy can help alleviate tension headaches. However, there are only a few clinical trials to support the use of trigger point therapy in the treatment of tension headaches.

Pain in the lower leg

A small study published in the Journal of Orthopaedic and Sports Physical Therapy in 2011 reveals that point therapy can help alleviate plantar heel discomfort.

For the purpose of the study, a total of 60 participants with plantar heel pain were divided into two groups: stretching was done by one, while trigger point therapy was done by the other (in addition to following the same stretching program as the first group). Point therapy resulted in a more significant improvement in physical function and a greater reduction in pain after one month.

Degenerative Diseases of the Nervous System

According to a pilot study published in the journal Movement Disorders in 2006, bringing about point therapy shows promise in the treatment of specific symptoms associated with Parkinson's disease.

For the study, 36 Parkinson's patients were treated with either trigger point therapy or music-based rest therapy twice weekly for a month before the results were tallied. Users of bring about point therapy showed a more significant improvement in engine performance at the conclusion of the trial. Despite both groups' moderate gains in quality of life, only those in the music rest group saw an improvement in their mood and stress levels.

How to Use Trigger Point Therapy

If you're considering trigger point therapy, ask your doctor for help locating a qualified practitioner.

It's too early to promote activation point treatment as a remedy for any ailment because of the lack of evidence. When it comes to treating a mental illness, it's important to realize that skipping or postponing conventional therapy might have major consequences. Consult a doctor if you're considering using induce point therapy for any medical reason.

Chapter 3

Benefits of Trigger Point Therapy

Neural markers are thought to be responsible for both the discomfort and benefits of activation point therapy. They are thought to be disrupted by activation point therapies. The goal is to alleviate discomfort while simultaneously teaching the muscles new, pain-free habits. Neuromuscular discomfort and inflammation can be lessened, flexibility can be increased, and adaptability and coordination can be improved in this way. In addition to lowering blood pressure, the procedure has been shown to boost circulation.

These include arthritis, carpal tunnel syndrome, chronic pain in the trunk, knees, and shoulder blades, migraines, menstrual cramping (including cramping during menstruation), MS, muscle spasms, stress, and weak spots, postoperative pain (including sciatica), tendonitis, and whiplash injuries.

Trigger point therapists are typically referred to by healthcare professionals. There will be a requirement for a brief history of any unintentional injuries that have occurred, as well as any hobbies or sports that you have participated in. She or he will ask the person in question for help in getting a detailed description of the pain and where it is coming from.

The therapist will conduct a thorough examination of the area around the trigger point. It is possible to provide lidocaine, saline, or other drugs by injecting them or by probing with a dry needle. For a long time, the therapist will apply sustained pressure to the spot with their fingers, knuckles, or elbows.

The effects of treatment might be felt almost immediately. Extend the muscles of your trigger point after an injection or pressure treatment. A final set of exercises is taught to the patient in order for their muscles to be better educated and for them to avoid experiencing pain in the future.

Trigger point therapy workbooks are available for patients to use at home in order to benefit from the therapy's self-treatment advantages.

Get Ready

To make sure the pain isn't being caused by a fracture or disease, patients should consult with a doctor before beginning active point therapy. A licensed induce point therapist will not treat a patient who has not been referred to them by another healthcare provider.

A padded table or treatment chair is typically used during the therapy process. Normal people should wear loose-fitting clothing that is comfortable for them. Classes will be made more effective by open communication between the student and the therapist.

Treatments range anywhere from 30 minutes to an hour. The average cost per program is between $45 and $60. *Acute pain* can be alleviated with just one application. Numerous treatments may be required for chronic pain.

Precautions

Point therapy should not be used on people who have recently been infected with a contagious disease or have recently been injured.

Bringing about point treatment can cause bruising in those using anticoagulant prescription drugs.

Research as Well as the General Public's Opinion

Activating point therapy has lately been the subject of some research because of the increased acceptance of acupuncture within the mainstream medical establishment.

One study by numerous Japanese experts found that the outcome of point therapy was superior to typical allopathic medications in relieving the pain of renal colic, indicating an increased interest in induced point therapy throughout Europe, Asia, and the United States.

It has been reported by the American Academy of Pain Management (AAPM) that trigger point therapy has been studied in small groups of less than ten people. In spite of the AAPM's efforts, point therapy has been accepted as a legitimate method of pain management and relief.

Trigger point therapy might be considered an addition to treatment in the original medical community. Psychiatrists, orthopedic cosmetic surgeons, and anesthesiologists are among the medical professionals who are familiar with their patients.

Chapter 4

How Trigger Point Therapy Works

As a result of muscle stress (*from accidents in cars or falls or sports or work-related accidents etc.*), postural stress from improperly standing or sitting for long periods at a computer, psychological stress (anxiety) and harmful toxins in the environment (allergies), trigger points may appear. If a trigger point isn't handled correctly, it can have ramifications for all of your other trigger points in the future.

The Causes of Pain

Your instinct is an attempt to protect yourself in the wake of a potentially hazardous "*event*." Changing how you move, sit, or stand can alter the load on your muscles, tendons, ligaments, and bones, causing them to fatigue. This results in muscle imbalances as well as postural problems throughout the body.

Your blood circulation may become limited, causing both your peripheral and central nervous systems to disseminate these "referred" pain indications, making evaluation and treatment even more difficult. Because of this, some experts believe that fibromyalgia may begin at induced sites. Is it possible for things to get much worse? Stay with it.

A good way to demonstrate how a single result in a muscle can cause back discomfort, sciatica, or a herniated disc is seen below. The Quadratus Lumborum (QL), a piece of low-back tissue right above the hips, is the most typical site for a trigger point. Regardless of what sets off the trigger point, your QL will weaken over time as it becomes increasingly shortened and tight.

The location of the pelvis will change as the QL gets increasingly dysfunctional. The abnormal curvature of the backbone caused by a malfunctioning pelvis will place an abnormal strain on the disc. The disc will begin to swell as time goes on. Within the context of your general standard of living, this is an example that will progressively worsen. Depression is a common follow-up.

Identifying Your Induce Points

If you have persistent discomfort, tightness, or limitations in specific tasks, there's a good likelihood that you're dealing with the effects of an induce point. Everyone has *"activation"* variables. It is possible that the same trigger can cause symptoms as varied as dizziness and numbness on one side of the body, as well as earaches and sinusitis on the other.

If you've ever had a headache because of a trigger point in the neck of your guitar or jaw, you'll know what I'm referring to. In the case of joint discomfort in the wrist, hip, leg, and ankle that is frequently misdiagnosed as arthritis, tendonitis, or ligament injury, they are the way to go. In the book *"Why We Harm: An Entire Physical & Religious Guide to Recover from Your Chronic Pain,"* by **Dr. Greg Fors**, the primary reason why a wide range of diseases are rooted

Additional signs and symptoms to be aware of include: restless leg syndrome (RLS), chronic toothache (TCP), plateaued exercise (TP), painful periods (TP), and irritable bowel syndrome (IBS).

An individual can't transform his or her cells by simply massaging the top layer of skin with a massage lotion, a vibrating massager, or by utilizing heat. The "knotted-up area" demands a long-term application of deep pressure.

There will be an increase in blood flow and a decrease in muscular spasm as the trigger point is worked on, as well as a break-up of scar tissue production. It will aid in the removal of any metabolic waste that may have accumulated.

It is also possible that the body will undergo a neurological release, lowering pain signals to the mind and resetting your neuromuscular system to its appropriate function. Simply put, everything will function properly once again.

Trying to Find Help

This is because the length of time you've been experiencing the trigger point affects how long it takes to release it. The number of activation factors you have, the effectiveness of your current treatment, and the frequency with which you can administer or receive treatment are all additional considerations.

The time and money it will take for your body to release all of its primary, latent, and myofascial trigger points, even if you're fortunate enough to find a practitioner who can do so correctly — let alone treat induce points — is time-consuming and pricey. Try a therapeutic massage, but bring about spots that are quite volatile; they must be dealt with daily using a technique that will administer the appropriate amount of pressure. It's unlikely that you'll be able to get a trigger point release via regular visits to a massage therapist.

A Methodology That Makes Sense.

Everything You Need to Know is Right There.

A trigger point is around the size of a mustard seed, which is one of the tiniest seeds in the world. The idea is to apply a sustained amount of stress to the area for a predetermined amount of time on a regular basis. In order to accomplish this, there are a wide range of methods available. Because of this, you'll need to think about taking the initiative.

Understanding how to deal with your musculoskeletal pain is essential, says **Dr. Simons**. It isn't just about short-term relief when it comes to dealing with myofascial trigger factors, which are the root causes of this type of pain. Your own active points are much easier to fix than anyone else's, and you may do so without a second thought. Dr. Simons' advice is spot-on: you need to keep up-to-date on your situation and then put what you've learned into practice. In today's world, the conventional wisdom is that if one of us is sick, the rest of us should seek you out so you can take care of the situation for everyone.

Taking Charge of Your Care

You may, of course, find yourself in need of medical attention at some point. However, the more you know, the better your treatment will be. You'll have to put in some time and effort, but the payoff will be quicker and the outcomes better.

Advice

Book an appointment with your doctor to make sure the issue isn't more serious. Many doctors are beginning to recognize the value of massage and may be able to prescribe it for you, allowing you to use your insurance or flex dollars to pay for it.

Chapter 5

How Will You Get a Result in Point Within Your Neck?

There are many mechanical causes that can generate trigger points, such as stress or strain on muscle tissue. *Trigger points* can be caused by a spinal injury, such as whiplash from a car accident or an injury sustained while participating in sports.

It's possible to foster the development of a trigger point by doing the same things every day for an extended period of time. For example, improper posture *(such as sleeping on an unsupportive pillow or craning your neck when using a computer)* or carrying a large handbag that puts undue strain on your neck, spine, and shoulders can cause neck and back pain.

How similar are trigger factors and tender factors to fibromyalgia?

There is a tendency for trigger points to be mistaken for fibromyalgia's soft components. Bring about points and sensitive elements are two types of localized pain, but they are not identical.

There is no direct link between tender variables and referred or spreading pain. Soft components in fibromyalgia are also symmetrical, appearing on both sides of the body. In an asymmetrical design, trigger factors do not appear.

This is where things become tricky, though: Fibromyalgia patients may experience both sensitive and resultant spots. Fibromyalgia sufferers may also have myofascial pain symptoms. As a result, it's critical to talk to your doctor about the specific methods for dealing with the various types of pain.

Why is it Difficult to Diagnose Trigger Factors?

Many types of back pain are caused by trigger factors, but doctors don't know as much as they should about how they work and how to treat them. Doctors don't have a clear concept of what causes pain points or any idea of how trigger variables cause symptoms to appear.

Trigger Factors Are Difficult to Define: They're both simple to identify but difficult to identify. They are capable of causing immediate and apparent muscle pain.

To make matters more complicated, they can take on the appearance of other issues. There is a tendency to mistake myofascial pain symptoms for fibromyalgia symptoms. A trigger point in the throat may cause jaw pain, earaches, or toothaches that don't go away completely.

Ask a doctor whether activating factors could be the source of your chronic throat pain if you don't know what it is. A physiatrist or other backbone specialist may be consulted by your doctor if he or she notices any abnormalities in your backbone, shoulders, or throat.

How to Treat Trigger Factors and Myofascial Pain Syndrome

There are several ways to treat trigger factors and myofascial pain syndrome, from simple home remedies to injections that your doctor must provide. When it comes to treating myofascial pain problems, there is no "magic" solution that works every time. In order to locate a remedy, you may wish to try a few things.

Therapeutic Interventions Performed in the Comfort of One's Own Home

The trigger point's discomfort can be excruciating, and you'll want to cure it at home as soon as possible. You should, however, see a trained specialist before beginning any at-home therapy so that you can diagnose the exact location of the problem and manage it efficiently.

In order to treat trigger points, you may need to massage the area, which might be difficult if they're located near your spine. As an alternative to using your hands, rolling over a baseball or rugby ball slowly and lightly can provide immediate relief.

Therapeutic Massage

Therapists proficient in deep tissue massage may be able to ease pain at a trigger point. Regular therapeutic massage treatments can help reduce the occurrence of myofascial pain symptoms and chronic trigger points.

Dry Needling

Injecting a bright needle and moving it around is how experts believe dried-out needling lessens activation point pain. If blood flow to the muscle is increased, this treatment could help lessen muscular contractions. It's possible that this treatment will help keep pain signals away from the actual site of the result, but additional research is needed to verify this claim.

Physical Therapy

Massage, heat, electric stimulation, and ultrasound are among the options available to physical therapists for treating trigger points. The trigger point area could also be chilled with a spray before specific stretches to relax and decrease the tight muscles are performed.

Medications

Myofascial pain has been treated with a variety of muscle relaxants. To avoid side effects, they should only be used in conjunction with a quality physical therapy program and only when absolutely necessary. Preventing the use of sedatives like Valium (diazepam) is a good idea because they can lead to addiction.

Induce Point Injections

Trigger point injections may be recommended by your doctor if you continue to experience myofascial pain symptoms despite following the therapy mentioned. In other words, your doctor may advise you to attempt less intrusive therapies like therapeutic massage first before moving on to injectable therapy, which is what these shots are thought to be for. When combined with a fitness or physical therapy regimen, injections can help you feel and perform at your highest level. Steroid medicines should not be injected, and these procedures should not be repeated. If you're looking to get the best results from these shots, you'll often only need a saline injection with a small amount of Procaine (also known as Novocaine).

Trigger Factors in the Throat

Inducing spots around the throat, which affect nearly everyone, remain a mystery when it comes to diagnosis and treatment. You can help prevent myofascial pain symptoms by training a proper posture and healthy vertebral technicians. A variety of therapies, such as therapeutic massage and physical therapy, can assist people with persistent trigger points manage their discomfort and get more out of their daily activities.

Chapter 6

Therapeutic Massage for Throat Pain, Upper Body Pain, Spine Pain etc.

The cantankerous scalene muscle group is located in the throat's private area, deep within the anatomical Bermuda Triangle. Massage therapists have gone missing while working in this enchanted location. Inexperienced massage therapists have a hard time dealing with the location and its muscles, which are complex and unique. Several joint pain problems in the throat, chest, arm, and spine can be alleviated by massaging the scalene muscles, and this short article describes how to do so. Scalenes are a challenging yet rewarding muscle group to work with!

Someone is holding a blade to the throat of the assailant. *"It's my hands,"* the caption states. *"My hands are sore,"* I *tell myself.* This is an example of some of the more odd forms of pain that can be caused by the scalenes.

In terms of muscle groups, the scalenes are unique. If your throat pain is persistent or severe, you might want to start with my advanced tutorial on throat pain.

Scalenes have been linked to a wide range of symptoms, including throat soreness and headaches, but this is just the beginning. The scalenes are a remote portion of the torso, and trigger points are more likely to be found in this location than in other muscle groups in the torso. Because of this oddity, the dominant mechanism is the perception of *"known pain."* Scalene pain can occur anywhere, but it is most commonly felt in the scales themselves. Instead of your scalenes, your upper body could be the problem.

In the shoulder and equip, for example, cardiac episodes can be felt, but the scalene muscles regularly produce exceptionally complex, adaptable, and significant patterns of recognized discomfort that are not found in any other type of muscle pain. Many people don't know that the scalenes can cause weird symptoms, even doctors and therapists.

Anatomical representation of the scalene muscle group's pain centers. Scalenes may play a role in upper body, spine, jaw, face, headaches, equipment, and hand pain, according to this illustration.

Creating a symphony of agony

Painful scalene muscles spread across the upper body, the spine and upper body, the hook and hands, and the medial side of the top, just like the discomfort of a cardiac attack. The pain described in the trunk may feel like a piercing stab going straight through the middle of the chest.

Additional intriguing (in the Chinese curse meaning) effects of scalene trigger points include those on your voice tone, swallowing, emotions, feelings that permeate the entire brain and sinuses, hearing, and teeth. I've observed scalene trigger points to be clinically extremely significant for diseases as seemingly unrelated as:

- A professional vocalist with an unexplained deterioration in his tone of voice *(aided by the release of scalene and other throat trigger points)*

- At least two patients who had surgery to try to correct severe chronic sinus infections *(one of these was practically cured by scalene activate point release alone, the other significantly cured).*

- There is a feeling of a lump in the throat even though there is no actual mass *("globus sensation")* due to the brachial artery and brachial nerve plexus being impinged by tight scales in the neck.

In other words, scalene-inducing factors are *"episode queens,"* with symptoms and effects that show in exorbitant proportion to the small and hidden muscles they influence. They are often a factor in other problems that take place in the region. Scalene Trigger points are like gangs in that they cause havoc in the community. There are numerous issues that can arise as a result of the anterior scalene.

Scalene Mythology

Maybe scalenes are not needed in the clinical setting. Many therapeutic massage therapists place certain muscles on an odd pedestal, making them the scapegoat for an exorbitant number of ailments. One of the most well-known examples of muscle mystique is the huge psoas muscle, located deep in the pelvis and stomach, but the scalenes muscle is perhaps the other prominent example, and they are physically identical.

Classic Gray

Other deep throat flexors include the scalenes.

Because there is so little substance to the "Perfect Places" talk about Psoas, I've omitted it from the series. Scalene buzzes, on the other hand, have a more substantial kernel of truth. True, many professionals exaggerate the significance of scalenes; however, there is some rational justification for this.

A group of deep cervical flexors, including the scalenes, form the bulk of the cervical flexors. To relieve a sore throat, many people are turning to exercises that target the throat's muscles. See? Strengthen your deep cervical flexors. The throat's "primary" conditioning

The Anatomy of Anatomical Bermuda Triangle

They fan out from the neck bone pieces, forming a rib cage that goes above the collarbone. *The anterior, middle, and posterior scalenes* are part of the scalene muscle group. They frequently apply to the very tops of the throat vertebrae and the topmost ribs at the very bottoms. Scalenes, on the other hand, are primarily used to pull the head to one side. Furthermore, despite the fact that they move the throat, they are also breathing and exhaling muscles because of the way they pull on the ribs.

To top it all off, the scalene muscles can extend all the way down between the ribs and attach directly to the very tops of some people's lungs, while in others, they can extend all the way down between their bones and attach directly to the very tops of other people's lungs. These are, in addition to the diaphragm, one of the few muscles that directly attach to the lungs. The pleura, the membrane that shrink-wraps the lungs, is where they pull through. Definitely a unique set of muscles! This degree of anatomical variation is actually rather common in human anatomy as a whole.

They are not difficult to find as a group, but the scalenes are complex in terms of their specifics. They fill the space between the triangle's three apparent constructions:

The Collarbone

The trapezius and shoulder muscles, lengthy V-shaped throat muscles *(sternocleidomastoid or, if that's too much of a mouthful, only the SCM),*

The scalene muscle group and optimum location No. 4 can be found where?

Somewhere in this triangle is Perfect Place 4. I assume that the most common clinically significant result point is in the stomach of the center scalene; this is the location that patients are most likely to feel is significant.

However, I don't like to set you on a wild goose chase after trying to identify exactly that spot. You should look around the triangle since you never know what you might find. It's not just the weather that's changing: One day, Perfect Place 4 may preserve a segment of the triangle, while the next, it may not. A desire to try is all that is required, not precise self-treatment.

With the recipient's face up, the best method to approach this is from the top. For those who don't have access to a massage table, it's helpful to focus on the part of the bed. It's important to keep your fingers smooth and place them in the hollow of the triangle, which is located just above your collarbone, just before the huge trapezius muscle, and just outside the conspicuous V-shaped sternocleidomastoid muscles of your neck.

The hands will be slightly angled inward and aimed at the sternum in this position. Using finger pads rather than fingers, press down and slightly inwards on the ropy muscles that fill the triangle. You don't have to worry about being too precise when you apply large amounts of force to trigger points and tense muscles.

Working your way around the triangle with your fingertips, gently strumming across the ropy muscular rings as a result, the area is a rich minefield of points, some of which will be beneficial and intriguing.

Risk!

It's possible to impinge on arteries or nerves in this location if you're careless, but it's not likely. For the love of all that is holy, don't use any kind of tool in this part of the body during massage therapy.

Cool down if you feel a pulse in your carotid artery or jugular vein. This is a bad place to rub. Rather than rubbing your eyeball, you forget about the need to rub the carotid artery in your neck. However, despite the fact that nerves can withstand far more pressure than the average person realizes and that smaller vessels aren't a problem, it may be foolish to take any chances in this field.

Is there anything more I should know? Trachea and the tone of the voice box are sensitive, but they are also too central for scalene therapeutic massage to be impeded by thoughtless pressure.

How Should Scalene Therapeutic Massage Make You Feel?

Some muscles respond better to massage than others. In general, therapeutic massage on the scalene is not particularly enjoyable. The throat is particularly prone to infection. Many people fear the pressure here, so don't underestimate it if you have any doubts about the safety of therapeutic massage or don't understand the strange feelings that are prevalent in this field. Avoid underestimating it. If the level of sensitivity is high, a great gentle method may feel hot and uncomfortable at first; this is not the type of trigger point you want to play with for fun. Wow, you've got my attention! Surely, it's a wonderful idea! However, the terrible news isn't all negative.

Scalene massage can be enjoyed right out of the box by some people, while others must "work through" it and become accustomed to its more unpleasant sensations before they can appreciate it. Assuming, of course, that your scalene muscles are under stress and causing a chronic pain problem, then it will feel like you've found the spot where you've been trying unsuccessfully to scratch an itch.

Your chances of having a positive experience are increased if you move gently and respectfully while massaging the scalenes with broad and less "poky" pressure. So much pressure can only produce the best scenario: a strange deep pain that spreads across the head, chest, and arms. Scalene therapeutic massage, at its best, appears difficult but "serious." Scalenes are elevated to a central role in the scene thanks to the dazzling suggestion patterns. "What the hell is that?" is a common response to seeing an entire body "lighting up" with visible pain after feeling a slight pressure in the throat. There is no other muscle that can elicit such jaw-dropping remarks.

Many individuals will exclaim, "Holy, the actual hell is that?" when they see a whole limb "lighting up" with visible pain from a light pressure in the throat. However, "certain activation factors are more the same than others" when it comes to the various types of pain. Even while massaging the scalenes can be painful at first, the benefits of this "perfect place" can be substantial over time.

Consequently, be prepared for everything and ease up.

You may have to "sort through" a little unpleasantness in order to get to the nicer feelings, but that's not impossible. There is no such thing as "no pain, no gain" in this business. There is a learning curve for patients in this sector. If you persist politely, it's possible that the sensation will change from hot to warm, from sharper to achier. It might only take a few days of bribing the area to make the switch, or it might take hours.

The amount of effort you should put in should be limited to what you can afford. If your time and work don't begin to shine after a reasonable amount of time, then this "perfect place" isn't really perfect and you should disregard it.

If you suffer from lateral epicondylitis, you're not limited to playing tennis.

The link between breathing and mood (theoretical but plausible)

Many joint problems and aches, particularly in the neck, upper back, and shoulders, may be caused in part by poor inhalation and exhalation. Even if it's just a theory, the connection between pain and breathing and exhaling is based on a simple principle: if the diaphragm doesn't do its job well, muscles in the upper chest and neck (sternocleidomastoid and scalenes) attempt to take over in order to compensate. Because these muscles aren't designed for regular breathing, they're prone to overwork and exhaustion, which can lead to pain and injury. From simple discomfort to more serious issues like rotator cuff and whiplash injuries, the consequences can be wide-ranging.

Additionally, unusual and cranky scalene muscles are likely to be the source of symptoms in this situation. Start seeing the Respiration Connection for more information.

The linkage

Because of this, if the diaphragm doesn't do a good job, other muscles in the chest and throat are forced to step in and do the work of the diaphragm if the diaphragm itself is dysfunctional. Unfortunately, these muscles aren't designed for automatic respiration, and as a result, they become fatigued and even injured.

Scalene overuse can occur as breathing becomes more difficult. There are various alternatives, but perhaps the most common and preventable is smoking, which is also a risk factor for chronic pain independently, so it's a combined whammy. However, this is simply a hypothesis, but smokers may have a greater number of trigger elements in their respiratory muscles that are more uncomfortable and persistent.

Scalenes and Lateral Epicondylitis Have an Unexpected Connection.

If the scalene's lateral epicondylitis relationship is anything to go by, it is a great example of how strange and clinically relevant the scalene really is.

Lateral epicondylitis, often known as lateral epicondylitis, is a common problem for typewriters and racquet sports players. It's often referred to as an inflammatory disorder, but it's not always that simple. Forearm muscles' Perfect

Place No. 5 myofascial trigger point is likely to play a significant role, independent of the presence or absence of lateral epicondylitis.

Furthermore, it appears that Perfect Place No. 4 has a considerable effect on Perfect Place No. 5. Forearm extensor digitorum points are typically treated with "scalene muscle induce points,". Trigger factors are located on the forearm's trunk. In this regard, the treatment of the Perfect Place number.

Chapter 7

Basic Self-Massage Methods for Myofascial Result in Points

Become adept at manipulating your own triggers (muscle knots). When it comes to self-massage, it may seem like a waste of time. Muscle "knots" or "cause factors": little patches of contracted muscle fibers that are delicate and cause soreness and stiffness are the most likely reasons to massage your muscles. In many common pain conditions, such as lower back and throat discomfort, they may play an important role. Most minor trigger points can be taken care of on their own.

Self-massage can provide greater relief from this type of tension than a massage practitioner can. Expert advice can be useful, but it may also be cost-effective to figure out ways of avoiding trigger variables. Self-help for most common pain issues can be done safely, cheaply, and effectively using this strategy.

- There is enough scientific debate about trigger factors to make it a contentious issue.It's evident that animals have issues with sensitive areas in our smooth tissue, but their nature is still unclear, and the popular belief that they may be some kind of mini-cramp could be erroneous. •. Even if massaging them has any effect, we have no idea. Pain can be treated experimentally with trigger point massage.

Trigger points can be treated with self-massage, and this explains the basics of doing so.

Why is it so easy to deal with little trigger points?

Self-massage with your thumbs or inexpensive instruments like a golf ball can ease a surprising amount of trigger point discomfort. As unpleasant as some of the factors may be, the bulk of them can be found and eliminated with only a little massage.

According to Dr. Janet Travell, self-massage is the cheapest, safest, and most effective way to alleviate the result of a point. This seems too wonderful to be true! As a result, we should presumably be skeptical. How does it happen that so little attention is paid to these issues?

The sensation of pain may become more of a phantom than a sign of tissue damage. Therapeutic massage may be able to help because there isn't much to "correct"—only a sensation to improve.

Small muscle knots can generally be treated with a little self-massage. However, how do these simple treatments actually work?

Perhaps, like stirring a stew to remove any lumps, stroking the muscles has a direct effect on building muscular mass. There is a theory that therapeutic massage works by pushing and draining waste materials, which theoretically pauses a vicious cycle and keeps the trigger point from returning, therefore preventing it from resurfacing. The problem is that, until now, no one has been able to demonstrate what kind of "knot" can be loosened by massage therapy.

Neurologically, isolated trigger sites are likely to be easier to manage. There is a far better possibility of solving the problem if it is limited to a single bodily part.

Trigger Point Self-Massage Instructions

For a basic case, a few mild massages may be all that is needed. If you're in a moderate scenario, a few days of massage for a few minutes at a time should be enough. Some of the most difficult situations that can be treated at home may necessitate an investment of up to six 5-minute treatments a day for a week. The problem is that none of these things are scientifically proven, and therapy will always fail.

Here are a few pointers:

What do you rub with? Use your fingertips, thumbs, fist, or elbow to rub the activation point. Whatever method works best for you, For locations that are difficult to access, simple instruments like balls and other accessible things are useful. The nutrients in golf ball massage therapy are unexpected! Using a foam roller, of course, would be beneficial, but the contact area is too large for most projects.

Pressure Positive's Backnobber, for example, can have a huge impact. A tennis ball, for example, may be found almost anywhere in the house and used for quick and easy self-massage as well.

In what way should I rub? Instead of worrying about the direction of the muscle fibers, simply perform short kneading strokes in either a round or backward and forward motion on the induce-point. Anything can happen. Stroke along the muscle fibers as though you're trying to lengthen them, because that could be more successful. However, it's occasionally obvious that muscle fibers have a distinct path.

How hard are you going to rub? This is just the beginning! Buying the right to improve your nervous system is an important part of therapeutic massage since it is mostly about using conversation with it. Helpful and friendly! instead of being obnoxious and impolite. As with Goldilocks, the technique should be exactly right: strong enough to fulfill, but easy enough to live with. You should aim for the 4–7 range on a scale of 10, with one being pain-free and ten being intolerable. When in doubt, go easy at first. Weak beginners tend to be overly enthusiastic. (Along with the experts!)

Is it going to be like this? When applying pressure to a muscle knot, it should be clear, robust, and satisfying; it should have a soothing, calming effect. When it hurts like that, you know it's good. Massage is like a conversation with your nervous system.

You'll also need the correct sculpt to get the job done. Helpful and friendly! Not obnoxious or impolite in the least. A milder approach is nearly always the best course of action. You need to be able to put your feet up. In the next section, you can learn more about the sensations you can expect from a therapeutic massage that achieves certain results.

What if something goes horribly wrong? It's unlikely, primarily because the pressure is balanced. Relieve yourself if you experience any side effects in the hours or days following therapy. A few days of daily treatment is enough time for cells to adjust to the more intense demands of vital therapy. Either the problem isn't trigger points, or these trigger points are much worse than you imagined.

What part of your body are you trying to rub? In the case of simple self-care, you can rely on your own instincts: just rub where it hurts! The epicenter of your symptoms is a good place to start looking for tender places, but you can limit your search to a relatively narrow area of muscle tissue. The greatest place to look for trigger factors, for example, is the top of your glenohumeral joint if you're experiencing pain in that area. The lump or "knot" in your muscle won't necessarily be felt by you, so don't worry about it.

The trigger point may not be where the pain is, but what if it is somewhere else? Bring in things that may cause symptoms that aren't where they're supposed to be. What should a novice do? This is the major outcome of point treatment, so don't worry about it too much. Do not worry about it unless important therapy is faltering. Remember the probability of misunderstanding recognized pain, but do not worry about it.

How much should you rub? Depending on how helpful it appears, therapeutic massage on each suspected spot for roughly 30 seconds. For most trigger factors, this is all you need! If rubbing the activation point is consistently elevating your mood, feel free to keep going for as long as you like-five minutes is about the maximum amount of time that any trigger point will require at one time.

How often do you rub? As long as you aren't experiencing any unpleasant responses, you should massage every trigger point that looks like it requires treatment at least twice a day, up to six times a day. More is most likely too exhausting and poses an unacceptably high risk of irritating it further.

Is there any way to tell if it's working? A little illustration of the thumb pressing down on the myofascial trigger point indicates "release," as shown in this image. For trigger points, self-massage is used to achieve a "release." What does it mean to "release" and how does it make you feel? Is there a way to assess your success? A weakening of the texture of the tissue, or "melting of the knot," is mainly what is observed here.

Although the phrase "release" is used, it does not have a precise scientific meaning. As a descriptor for the unknown, it refers to whatever happens when the trigger point disappears. In other cases, it may indicate that the strongly clenched muscle fibers are resting (or have been violently disrupted). It's also possible that it's just a "sensory" version that does nothing but halt the injury, or that it's insignificant and short-lived (like scratching a mosquito bite).

This could go unnoticed for some time. Cells may remain "polluted" with waste product metabolites even after a recent release, making things seem even worse until they get better. One theory suggests that the release of muscular knots may necessitate some damage to the knots' tissue. Because of this, even if you succeed, the area is likely to be extremely sensitive.

Initially, there is a satisfying yet intense impression of scratching an itch; nevertheless, the tissue is actually more sensitive thereafter, not less. Both are treated and being treated.

In the beginning, don't worry about the details; simply activate the point and trust that you've accomplished some sort of release, even if it's only partial; after that, wait for the trigger indicator to slow down and see what happens. If you were successful, you would see a big difference in your symptoms the next day.

As soon as the next morning, if you were successful, you would notice a significant decrease in your symptoms. Is it possible to have a good headache? If you use natural inducers, you're more likely to experience "pleasant pain"—a strong, satisfying feeling that is both painful and relieving. Even though it's not pleasant, the body "knows" and "wants" a lot of pressure, so it's a positive experience in the same way barfing is. A trigger point release is far more likely if you are experiencing "good pain."

If, on the other hand, you're grimacing or wincing, you should probably be kinder. For many patients, therapy success depends on their level of comfort. You're too harsh on yourself, especially in the early phases, if you can't massage the result without wailing. It's not uncommon for a trigger point to feel like it's on fire, but it still releases. Such a rotting trigger point, on the other hand, may require more extensive or long-term treatment. When it comes to the "pressure question," it's surprisingly difficult to answer.

This is just the tip of the iceberg when it comes to Trigger points.

Basic self-massage can go wrong for a variety of reasons. It's possible that the doubters are correct; perhaps all that's there is a strange sensation and nothing in the body to fix. Because of a neurological condition known as "referred pain," the Trigger point may not be located in the exact location where the pain is felt. As a result, people find up going on wild goose hunts and rubbing things they don't need to be rubbing. In addition, there are many more of them, designed specifically for circumstances where space is limited.

Chapter 8

Neck Muscle Knots

You could strum your neck muscles like guitar strings if they weren't so tense. This tune, on the other hand, is not for the faint of heart. Is massaging, pressing, and probing actually assisting it in healing? On the other hand, wouldn't you be contributing to the problem?

Your stiff muscles might start singing a happy tune if you follow a few simple instructions. Chad Adams, DC, a chiropractor, explains trigger point massage in detail:

Muscle knots: *A muscle freak-out*

Once again, your back and throat are in knots due to muscle knots caused by overwork and lack of sleep. They're also known as "trigger points," and they refer to tense spots in the muscle that won't let go.

"It's an indication from the mind that something is wrong, so I'm going to panic and get tense," explains Dr. Adams. "A result in point is a muscular spasm." Trigger factors are characterized by a series of recursive actions. For most of us, that's like swinging a rugby racket or hunching over our desks and banging the keyboard day after day, week after week.

While our bodies are built to handle a lot of stress, "we weren't meant to do the same thing every day," he explains. "Those few spots are calls for rescue," says the author.

It's unclear how to calm down the muscles that are on edge. I recommend starting with a self-massage technique known as a "trigger point," which involves pressing on the knots in the muscles. Muscles can be helped to relax by natural pressure.

For self-massage, here's how:

- If you're looking for a tight spot, it's likely you won't have to look far.

- Press forcefully into the trigger points with your fingertips (or tools like foam rollers and therapeutic massage balls).

- Repeat for 3 to 5 minutes at least five or six times a day, preferably more frequently.

What's the level of difficulty of the event you're driving to? It differs from person to person. Some people can handle a lot of stress, while others can't handle it at all (no shame). I think you won't cause any harm if you continue to press in.

Even so, it's not going to feel wonderful right away. I explained that "pain is the area of the procedure." Extreme pain, on the other hand, is not. If you feel a painful pinch or tingling, you probably have a personal injury that extends beyond muscle tension. If so, stop using your thumbs and see a doctor immediately. Make a major difference in your surroundings. Refuse to give up.

Each mini-massage should loosen the muscles. Regular trigger point massages can help relieve pain for extended periods of time.

However, you should also think about how you might improve your surroundings to make your muscles happier. Is it possible that a much better desk chair could help your situation? No, breaks aren't allowed during the workday.

If you've already made the necessary adjustments and the knots keep reappearing, it's time to call in the experts. If you need help, see a chiropractor, physical therapist, or massage therapist.

Chapter 9

Chronic Throat Pain: What Condition is Leading to Throat Pain?

There are a wide range of conditions that can cause discomfort in the neck. The glenohumeral joint, the head, the equipment, and the hand might also be affected by discomfort in the neural pathways. The discomfort in the spinal cord can spread to the legs and the area below the throat, making it difficult to breathe.

Types of Throat Pain

In most situations, neck discomfort will go away after a few days or a few weeks, but if the pain lingers for weeks, it may be indicative of a more serious medical condition. Sometimes, early action may be necessary to achieve the best outcome.

Diagnosis and Treatment Options for Neck Pain

There are several ways that a sore throat can hurt:

- A stiff neck that makes turning the hat difficult.

- A single point of stabbing or razor-sharp pain.

- A general sense of unease or sensitivity

- Radiating pain in the shoulders, arms, or fingertips, as well as pain radiating up into the head, are all examples.

In some cases, other symptoms like the following may be a symptom of neck discomfort:

- Tingling, numbness, or weakness that extends into the shoulder, hands, or fingers

- The difficulty of lifting or gripping a thing, etc.

- Walking, stability, or coordination issues

- Inability to regulate one's bowel or bladder function.

When is a Stiff Throat Serious?

The pain in the neck of the guitar may be minor and easily overlooked, or it may be so agonizing that it interferes with everyday activities, such as sleep. In some cases, the discomfort may be short-lived; in others, it may be continuous. It is possible that a patient's discomfort in the neck may be a symptom of a more serious condition, such as meningitis or cancer.

Straining or spraining of the neck can lead to cervical spine disorders.

What can go wrong with the cervical spine?

As a result, the cervical spine, or neck, is tasked with supporting and moving the top, which may weigh up to 11 pounds—the weight of a medium bowling ball.

Treatment for Throat Pain

Non-surgical techniques, self-care at home, and medical aid are the most common ways to treat throat pain.

Treatment of Throat Pain on One's Own Neck pain that isn't debilitating or the result of trauma can usually be treated on one's own. Throat pain can be treated at home in a variety of ways, including the following:

- **Relax:** If you have a strained or sprained throat, take a few days off from work. The muscles and tendons will heal on their own. You must exercise caution when engaging in activities or actions that cause pain.

- **Ice and warmth:** Inflammation and pain may be reduced by applying snow as an anti-inflammatory. First, applying ice or cold packs to the sore throat is a good idea since they can temporarily shut down tiny arteries and prevent the soreness from worsening. Snow or temperature might be used on an alternating basis after a few days. Inflammation can be exacerbated by using a high temperature on a regular basis.

- **Massage**: After administering cold or warmth, a therapeutic massage can ease muscle stress and spasms, thus lowering pain.

- **Better posture:** If your throat pain is caused by poor posture, making a few small adjustments to your posture may be the best treatment. Workstations that are more ergonomically friendly, such as one that has an adjustable desk and chair with an ergonomic display and keyboard, or one that allows you to rest on your back rather than on your stomach, can help keep your body, head, and throat in an all-natural posture as you work.

- **Modify your lifestyle:** If certain activities cause recurring throat pain, you may want to reduce or discontinue them. Texting buddies while craning your neck to see the screen is a bad habit that needs to be curbed. The phone should be placed closer to your eyes so that you can see what you're typing while you're texting.

- **Over-the-counter medications:** There are a variety of over-the-counter drugs available that can either reduce swelling or block the transmission of pain signals to the brain. There is a danger in using these drugs without proper caution. Avoid overdosing by reading all the instructions and cautions on the label of the pain medicine. For example, acetaminophen, the active ingredient in Tylenol, is also included in many other common medications, such as those used to treat the common cold and allergic reactions.

Throat Pain Treatment without Surgery

Non-surgical methods, such as you or a combination of the following, are commonly used in the treatment of some types of neck pain:

- **Physical therapy**: Most treatment plans include some physical therapy to improve neck strength and flexibility. Based on the diagnosis and situation, the physical therapy program's framework and length will be different. There will be a lot of physical therapy for the first few months. After that, the patient will be able to do their own exercises at home.

- **Pain relievers:** If an over-the-counter remedy does not work, prescription-strength pain relievers can be tried. There are a wide variety of pain drugs on the market, each with its own set of risks and advantages. The CDC changed its recommendations in 2016 and urged fewer opioid prescriptions for chronic pain management because of the danger of addiction and other probable problems. The CDC had previously recommended opioids as a common treatment.

- **Cervical epidural steroid injections**: A cortisone steroid solution is injected into the exterior coating of the vertebral canal, the epidural space, in order to alleviate pain. Fluoroscopy (X-ray help) can be utilized to ensure that the injection moves into the epidural area near the inflamed nerve. The injection's goal is to reduce the effect of a disc herniation on nearby nerves or tissues. These injections can ease the patient's discomfort so that he or she can resume normal activities and progress with physical therapy. This injection has some risks, including the possibility of infection, and its usage may be restricted to a few times a year, if not prohibited altogether.

- **Cervical facet injections:** Steroid injections into specific bones in the neck can alleviate throat pain caused by discomfort in the facet vital joints. Radiofrequency ablation (RFA) of the facet's important joints' tiny sensory nerves may be recommended if facet shots yield predictable but short-term results. When it comes to the long-term effects of these RFA treatments, these shots are just meant to provide temporary relief for the aching facet bones.

- Pain can be obtained by causing discomfort to certain muscle bundles through **trigger point injections**. In order to restore the normal orientation of the irritated muscle bundles, point injections are administered. Injections other than saline, lidocaine, dextrose, or cortisone may be administered. For throat muscular irritations with clearly identified activation points, this treatment may be complex but persuasive. In other cases, these treatments may not be long-lasting or provide the necessary pain-reduction.

- In order to increase the range of motion and alleviate discomfort, a chiropractor or other medical professional may perform **manual manipulations** on the backbone. Manual manipulation, also known as chiropractic adjustment, is typically performed on a desk in an office setting. In most cases, the adjustments are performed by the chiropractor's hands, but a machine may be utilized to make minor adjustments. There is some evidence that chiropractic realignment can help alleviate symptoms of throat pain, but not everyone agrees. High-velocity cervical backbone modifications have also been linked to undesirable outcomes such as heart attacks or paralysis, although this is rare.

- **Acupuncture**: With roots in Chinese medicine dating back hundreds of years, acupuncture involves inserting thin needles at the body's tips to treat a variety of ailments. The needles are often withdrawn after less than an hour of treatment. Reusing needles is not permitted in the United States. You should only use sterile needles and a qualified acupuncturist for your treatment. Most patients tolerate acupuncture well, and it is generally thought to be safe.

It's important to note that this list doesn't include every conceivable treatment for neck discomfort.

Neck discomfort can be reduced in the long run by a variety of methods, including the ones listed above as well as healthier lifestyle choices made by the typical individual. For example, a moderate amount of aerobic movement several times a week, as well as the avoidance of smoking, is a good strategy for most throat ailments.

C h a p t e r   1 0

How to Relieve Throat Pain with Acupressure

Neck pain is frequently caused by tension in the muscles and the strain on the back. It's also possible that worn and split cartilage in key joints is a contributing factor. Throat pain tends to be concentrated in a single area of the throat, but it can also spread out. Tightness or spasms may be necessary to deal with this type of discomfort.

Reflexology and acupressure have long been used to treat neck pain. Acupressure is a way of massaging and activating certain points on the body in an effort to help people with different types of health problems.

Reflexology's clinical performance is still being tested, but anecdotal information suggests that it works for many people. By reading on, you can learn more about the various factors that may alleviate your pharyngitis.

Neck Pain and Pressure Points: The Scientific Basis

An acupuncture treatment for throat discomfort has been widely researched and is considered a reliable source of information. Acupressure for throat pain isn't universally acknowledged because there is some evidence that acupuncture works. The use of acupuncture needles raises the question of whether or not the body's own healing chemicals are triggered by the procedure. If this is the case, then using massage instead of needles to stimulate pressure factors will not provide the same treatment.

Acupuncture, on the other hand, should not be ruled out as a holistic treatment for throat pain. It is possible to alleviate throat pain and aching muscles by reinvigorating pressure forces. The answer is that no one knows, according to a number of reliable evaluations of medical textbooks.

Factors Affecting Throat Pain

Follow these steps to try acupressure on your neck:

- Take a deep breath in and out. When performing acupressure treatments, be sure to do so in a peaceful and private location.

- To relieve your throat pain, apply firm, deep pressure to the pressure points you've identified using a massage stick. For best results, spend 3 to 4 minutes at each location, rotating your fingertips in an up-and-down or round-and-round motion. Stop the treatment immediately if you notice a sharp increase in discomfort anywhere in the body.

- If you believe the therapeutic massage therapy is effective, give it another go later in the day. With acupressure, there's no limit to how many times a day you can perform it.

The following is a list of pressure spots that can be used to alleviate various throat pains. Recognize that the whole individual is interrelated in reflexology. You may find yourself using one portion of the body as a way to activate or align a different one.

Jian Jing.

Jian Jing is located in the neck muscles, halfway between the base of your skull and the tips of your fingers. According to reliable sources, acupuncture studies of headaches and muscle tension have revealed this to be true. Sore or swollen throats can be efficiently treated by Jian Jing. If you're pregnant, don't use this method to reduce neck pain because it could lead to labor.

He Gu (L14)

The "web" fold of skin in the center of your thumb and fingers is where the He Gu point is located. Reflexologists claim that stimulating this area helps alleviate pain in a wide range of places, including the throat. Avoid reviving this point if you're pregnant.

Blowing wind Pool (Feng Chi/GB20)

It is located behind your earlobe, towards the top of your throat and the bottom of your head. It is called Feng Chi (GB20). From tiredness to headaches, reflexologists use this method. It is possible to alleviate a sore throat caused by sleeping in an awkward position by releasing this pressure point.

(TE3) Zhong Zhuang

You can find the Zhong Zu point between your pinky and ring fingers, just above your knuckles. When this pressure point is activated, it may stimulate numerous parts of the human brain, resulting in increased blood flow and a reduction in stress. Pressure or stress on the guitar's neck can be alleviated by stimulating this area.

Heaven's Pillar

Both sides of your neck, at the base of your head and two inches from where your backbone begins, have access to this area. This is where your shoulders meet your elbows. Inflammation of the lymph nodes and congestion from trusted source might cause a sore neck if this feature is stimulated.

Acupressure Factors for Neck Treatment

Hiren Acupressure

Acupuncture is an excellent method for relieving neck pain and throat tightness. There are a number of acupressure points on the neck that can be used in treatment. Pain and tightness in the throat are common occurrences today. A variety of approaches, such as medication, acupressure, and acupuncture, can alleviate throat pain and tightness. Acupuncture for Throat Pain Relief is included in this acupressure technique.

Tightness in the neck and shoulders, stress, and many other aches can be alleviated with acupressure factors for neck pain. Acupressure Factors has no side effects, which is the most important thing. Using acupuncture factors to treat neck pain from playing the guitar is completely safe. Acupuncture can be used to treat throat pain without causing any negative side effects.

Pain can be reduced, the disease can be stopped, or the body can hit back using acupressure. Simple to apply, acupressure factors provide speedier relief from throat pain and glenohumeral joint pain when applied repeatedly with the appropriate pressure. Acupressure points are located throughout the body in the following locations:

- Acupressure points on the neck.

- Acupressure points at the back of the neck.

- Acupressure points on the Head.

- Acupressure points on Shoulder Back.

- Acupressure points on Face.

When it comes to acupressure, the back of the head, shoulder back, and face are all areas that can benefit from it.

In cases of throat pain and tightness, acupuncture factors can help alleviate the discomfort. Throat pain's pressure factors can be summarized as follows:

- Acupressure Factors on the neck backside

- Acupressure Factors for Neck Pain

Some people find relief from throat discomfort and headaches by focusing on neck backside factors. A total of six throat rear acupressure points can be found on the backside of the throat. Heavenly Pillars, Heavenly Gates, and Heavenly Pillar Throat Backside Factors are divided into three sections: Let's take a look at each of these in turn:

Gates of Awareness:

In the back of your throat, you'll find the Gates of Awareness. The Acupressure Gates of Awareness Factors can be found in the void between the muscles in your throat. Perpendicular to the throat, the backside muscles are the pressure factors located at the base of the skull. As depicted in the image, the Gates of Awareness can be found.

The back of your neck at the Gates of Consciousness can be pressed with firm pressure to relieve neck pain, stiffness, irritation, dizziness, migraines, and other symptoms.

For Neck Pain: Acupuncture Factors

Throat backside points are influenced by the home window of Heaven. The Heaven Acupressure Factors for Throat Pain screen is positioned on the backside of the throat, next to the Gates of Awareness and below the bottom of the skull. In the notch at the base of the skull, Windows of Heaven Factors can be found. Take a look at these Windowpane of Heaven Factors:

If the Home Window of Heaven Factors is active on a regular basis, it can help you alleviate symptoms such as neck pain, a tight throat, glenohumeral joint pain, and headaches.

The Heavenly Pillar of Neck Backside Factors has two pressure factors. Underneath the skull's foot, there are

Heavenly Pillar Factors. The Heavenly Pillar Acupressure Factors are located around 2-3 cm below the base of the skull. As indicated, locate and apply pressure to the Heavenly Pillar pressure factors with your hands (or other implements).

The Heavenly Pillar is under stress. If you frequently practice Acupressure Factors, your insomnia, weariness, stiffness in the neck, and other symptoms of burnout and stress can be alleviated. Neck Pain and other neck-related issues can be alleviated more quickly and effectively by stimulating acupressure points on the back of the neck as part of a regular daily regimen.

A crucial acupressure site for neck pain is the back of the mind point. Acupressure In the exact back of your mind, you'll find the Back Again Mind Point. The Wind Mansion is located on the other side of the hand point. At the bottom of the skull is where Head Point is located. Once again, locate the acupressure point at the back of the mind, as depicted in the image below.

You can reduce neck pain, eye-ear pain, pain in the nasal area, stiffness in the neck, throat trouble, and back pain by frequently applying firm pressure on the acupressure point at the back of the top point.

Acupuncture Factors for the Back of the Neck and Shoulders:

These factors are quite helpful in alleviating stress and pain in the shoulder area. The glenohumeral joint collection of 3 centimeters is where the acupressure shoulder back factors are located, not in the lower neck. Make WellPoint is another name for the glenohumeral joint's back point. Find the exact location of the acupressure Glenohumeral joint back still point and apply gentle pressure to alleviate any discomfort. Below is a picture of Make Back Factors.

- Acupressure on the glenohumeral joint back factors, applied on a daily basis, can alleviate symptoms such as pain, weariness, glenohumeral joint tension, irritation, and more.

- Use extreme caution: if the woman is pregnant, do not apply pressure to the glenoid joint.

Acupressure Factors on the Face in Therapeutic Massage and Spa

When it comes to relieving throat pain, Face Factors are the best. This is where the Throat Pain Acupuncture Face Factors are located: under the eyebrows, on the bridge of the nasal area. Drilling bamboo is also known to have risk factors for throat pain. Face Point is located at the exact point where the bridge between the nose and the brow meets. According to the illustration, the following are the acupressure factors for throat pain:

There are several ailments that can be helped by the daily application of pressure to the acupressure face factors for neck pain.

Hand Factors can Reduce Throat Pain and Tightness in Throat Acupressure Points. Two separate acupressure points on the hands have been found to help alleviate throat pain with acupressure. It is possible to locate the First Hands Point by looking at your index and middle fingers. Start to see the picture displayed below to find the exact spot for First Hands Point. In your daily routine, apply light pressure to the first hand point, which helps alleviate throat pain and neck tightness.

The second hand point for throat pain is located near the end of the smallest finger (pinky). There is a specific acupressure point beneath the little finger. Find the pressure point, as illustrated in the image below, and press on it. Putting your hands on the Hands Indicate can help relieve throat pain.

Throat and Pain Acupressure: The Six Most Important Factors to Consider

The throat is a vital component of the human body, and although the brain is located in the head, it is the throat that has the ability to convert it in whatever way it chooses. Even if we're more likely to be afflicted by pain and aches in our throats and necks because of our more computer-centric lifestyles, we're also more likely to suffer from agonizing headaches. Reflexology can be used efficiently to provide long-term relief from anguish and terrible discomfort in the upper and throat areas since all of the points located there are yang elements, with extreme energy circulation through them.

Acupressure Can Treat Pain in the Throat and Glenohumeral Joints.

Causes of Throat and Mouth Pain:

Many things can cause our necks and shoulders to be stiff and painful, from simple things like sleeping in the wrong position to more serious things like arthritis and meningitis, all of which can leave us with a hurting and aching neck for days at a time.

Massages for the neck

- Poor sitting posture

- Poor sleeping posture.

- A pulled muscle

- Overexertion

- Sprain.

- Pains and aches in the neck.

A few days of stiffness and numbness in the neck and shoulder area are common, but they can be easily alleviated with a few simple exercises. When the pain in the throat persists for days or weeks, it can radiate to the shoulders, the back, and even the brain, depending on how severe the condition is.

Arthritis (Cervical spondylitis and rheumatoid arthritis) and **Meningitis** (Inflammation of the meninges surrounding the brain) are two major causes of neck and shoulder discomfort.

Such situations necessitate the prompt involvement of medical professionals.

Soothing Throat and Shoulder Aches with Acupressure

Pain in the glenohumeral and cervical joints can be debilitating and prevent us from going about our everyday lives, but reflexology can help us treat the problem from the inside out, leading to better overall health and mental peace.

Acupuncture can help you get rid of neck and shoulder pain.

A vital component of modern life's throbbing aches and pains is treated with acupressure, an ancient eastern recovery art with roots in traditional acupressure techniques. It can assist us in reducing anxiety and regaining a sense of equilibrium in our lives. Activating these six basic acupressure variables can be done by yourself, or someone you care about can benefit from a restorative acupressure program.

Shoulder Region: The shoulder joint is located half-way between your throat's foot and the glenohumeral joint's end on the humerus muscle. Reduced throat and shoulder stiffness can be achieved by focusing on this area. In addition, it aids in the alleviation of back discomfort.

In the occipital ridge, beneath the SCM muscle, lies the completion bone; this aspect is located in the depression behind the hearing. It helps alleviate headaches, throat discomfort, and dizziness by revitalizing this spot.

Neck Region: The occipital ridge, where the backbone enters the skull via the tendon, is where Heaven's Pillar appears on the neck. Neck pain, numbness, and tightness can be relieved by rubbing this point. Chronic cough can be reduced by revitalizing this area.

Head Region: Another section of the head consists of seven points. Figures 1–7, starting with the forehead, have been used to depict these elements in the schematic. The simultaneous activation of all of these mechanisms aids in the relief of arthritis-induced neck pain and frontal headaches.

Side Throat Region: Underneath and somewhat backward of the earlobe is where you'll find this feature. The stiffness in the throat and shoulders, as well as headaches, can be relieved by stimulating this spot.

Between your thumb and index finger, there is a valley called Union Valley. Stress and tension in the neck and shoulders can be relieved by rubbing this spot. Anxiety and stress can be relieved by reinvigorating this component.

Hands: You've learned about the specific acupressure sites that can be stimulated to alleviate the discomfort in the throat and improve the area, so here are some simple recommendations that you can utilize to help make the program an unforgettable experience for the recipient.

8 Simple Methods for a Productive Acupressure Session

You now know which acupressure spots to target to relieve throat discomfort and make the area feel better, so here are a few pointers for making the program a memorable one for the audience.

- Determine the source of the receiver's problem.

- Begin the acupressure session by instructing the recipient to stretch.

- Make the receiver lie down on a fresh mat.

- Pillows and towels, as well as other necessities, should be readily available.

- When you're not on the mat, use wrapped towels or clean clothes for support.

- By gently pushing on the components with your fingertips, you can ask if the pressure makes him/her feel good.

- Pressure should be applied simultaneously to the same variables on both sides of your body.

- Concentrate your attention on one area for two to three minutes before moving on to the next.

Acupressure has a long and distinguished history of application in the treatment of a wide range of ailments. It's comforting to feel the intense therapy enter your body and restore your body and the natural components to their proper balance. Don't forget to bring up your experience with using reflexology to treat neck discomfort.

Chapter 11

Trapezium Pain

Trigger points are frequent in the trapezius, causing transferred pain. Trigger points are the most common reason for patients to visit a doctor's office. The trapezius is a large, kite-shaped muscle that covers a large portion of the lower back and the back of the neck. The upper, middle, and lower trapezius muscles all have distinct functions and cause joint symptoms.

Common Symptoms of Trapezium Pain

Trapezium pain symptoms include frozen glenohumeral joint activities and myofascial dysfunction.

Upper Trapezius

Face, temple, or jaw pain; dizziness or vertigo (associated with the sternocleidomastoid muscle); severe neck pain; stiffness of the neck; lack of mobility; intolerance to weight on the shoulders.

Middle trapezius

Back pain; headaches near the base of the skull. " A nagging discomfort in the very top of the shoulder, near the joint, is associated with trigger point # 2; with trigger point # 6, it is associated with a burning sensation near the spine.

Lower trapezius

- pain in the neck, throat, or upper back

- There may be a similar referral pattern to the stratus posterior superior in that the pain may originate on the back of the shoulder blade, go down the inside of the arm, and end in the ring and little fingers.

- Trapezius Activate Point Images.

- Induce Point Therapy at Home Freezing to Make. Causes Exercise Treatment for Iced Shoulder.

- Rotator Cuff Muscle Exercises Tendonitis.

Causes and Perpetuation of Induce Points

There is a hemipelvis (the portion of the pelvis you sit on) that is smaller than normal. Short upper arms (which in turn causes you to slim down to one aspect to use the armrests)

Large breasts, fatigue, tense shoulders, cradling a phone between your ear and shoulder, a seat without armrests, typing with a keyboard, sewing on your lap with your hands unsupported, jogging, sleeping on your back or front with your mind rotated to the side for an extended period, playing the violin, athletics involving sudden one-sided movements, sitting with your arms crossed, all of these things contribute to the development of large breasts and large breasts alone (seated slumped).

Backpacking, biking, kayaking, and any other activity that necessitates a lot of bending over (such as working in electronics, dentistry, architecture, or as a draftsperson or secretary).

Overly tight bra straps (either the band or the torso strap).

It's not just carrying a heavy daypack or backpack that can cause harm to your joints; it's also doing so because of the risk of whiplash (from a car accident, falling on your head, or any other sudden jerk of the head), walking too slowly with a cane, and focusing your attention on just one part of the trail for too long.

Techniques and Hints

Consult a physician if you have short or asymmetrical upper arms so that you can have compensated elevates or pads. Modify or replace your furniture that doesn't fit. If your table is too far away from you, you won't be able to get low fat against the backrest. While working, keep your elbows relaxed on the surface of your project or on armrests at the same height. The armrests should support your elbows and forearms evenly. Your computer display should be in front of you with a copy attached to the medial side of the screen, so that you can always keep your eyes focused on the task at hand.

As a draftsman, engineer, or architect, you'll benefit from a tilted work table, but you'll need to take frequent pauses to avoid mechanical stress in a specific area.

Get a headphone or speakerphone for your mobile phone, or hold the phone in one hand while using it. Shoulder rests aren't sufficient. Make sure your bras fit properly. If, after removing your bra, you can see the elastic signs on your skin layer, the straps are too limited. Running bras are most beneficial to women with medium and small breasts.Ask the salesperson for help in locating a bra that is the right fit; most of them are knowledgeable about the products they sell.

Get rid of your foam rubber cushion! These pillows' vibrations will exacerbate the results of several factors. It's important that your pillow provides enough support for your mind while you are laying down to work (not too much or too brief). When I travel, I usually bring my travel pillow with me. I know that I have a pleasant place to relax, and that it will come in handy and be easy to get caught at an airport with it.

Insurance companies may pay for breast reduction surgery if your doctor recommends it because of big breasts that are causing you back pain. If you're considering surgery, be aware of the potential hazards.

Wear your daypack over both shoulders, with the straps crossing in front of your chest. Make sure your purse has an extended strap and is placed diagonally across your torso by putting the belt over your head and keeping the material light.

Put most of your weight on your hip strap if you're going backpacking. Trigger points can be caused and perpetuated by a head-forward posture, so correcting the position of the head is essential. When sitting in a car, at a table, in front of a PC, or even when eating dinner or watching television, a head-forward posture might be made worse. Every time you sit down, make sure your lumbar area is properly supported. 18. Begin by watching the video below to learn how to improve your posture.

Take frequent breaks if you have to sit for long periods of time. Setting a timer in the room will force you to get up and gently turn it off.

Make eye contact with the person you're talking to instead of focusing your thoughts on them. The trapezius muscle is required to put your hands in your pockets when you are standing up. Using many layers of glenohumeral joint pads helps alleviate the pressure on the upper trapezius.

Patients with occipital neuralgia and cervicogenic headaches who have not found relief from their symptoms through self-help methods such as activating points should seek medical attention. An examination by an osteopathic doctor or a chiropractor may reveal vertebrae that are misaligned.

Self-Improvement Methods

Recommendations for using these self-help approaches are detailed in the CD-manual. ROM's Click here to place your order. Please be advised that if you don't follow the CD-correct ROM's advice, you could make your discomfort worse.

Applying Pressure

Lay on your back with your legs bent, either on a corporate bed or on the ground. Start with a golf ball or racquetball and apply pressure for eight seconds to one minute at a time at the mark, about one in and out of the spine. Keep the pressure on each region by squeezing a little bit deeper into the tree trunk. Continue until you get to the rib cage's lowermost portion (the video demonstrates heading entirely to the very best of the pelvis, but also for the trapezius, you merely need to visit underneath the rib cage). If your back is broad or there are soft components further out, you might be able to continue performing this on another line further right out of the spine. This should almost never be done near the spine.

Lift the weight of your equipment by placing your elbow and forearm on a surface that is high enough to support it. Pinch the upper section of the trapezius muscle with the opposite hand, tilting your head slightly toward the side you'll be working on. Don't dig your thumb into the indentation above the collar bone and stick it to the flesh of the tissue.

The upper trapezius can also benefit from self-help exercises for the supraspinatus muscle. Place a rugby ball in the groove of a doorjamb while standing in a doorway and steadily storing the ball with your opposite hand. Repeat as necessary. Bend at about 90 degrees, and make sure your thoughts are completely relaxed! Use as much or as little pressure as you like to sink your teeth into the ball. As long as you're holding the ball in your opposite hand and your mind is calm, work the areas on the shoulder's surface.

Use a baseball and place it face up with your hands behind your neck to focus on the trunk of your neck. The baseball should be in the center of the best palm (not where the fingers sign up for the palm!) with one hand on top of the other. As a means of exerting pressure, focus your thoughts on the ball (do not place the ball on the backbone but the muscles aside from the spine). If you want to work on the medial side of the ball, move your head away from it and rotate your mind back to the medial side of the ball. If you want more pressure, rotate your account to the medial side, where you will be working more, and if you want less pressure, rotate your mindless.

Picking yourself up to go to the ball is not something you usually do. The muscles may feel more strain as a result. Revolving your head away from the ball is an excellent way to keep the ball in motion. From the base of the skull to the base of the throat, and from there, it is possible to reach the glenohumeral joint at the bottom of the throat.

Exercises

Swimming is a great way to build aerobic fitness without putting too much stress on your muscles. By varying your strokes, you can avoid putting undue strain on your trapezius muscles.

Thinking about something specific, such as the crawl heart stroke, can aggravate your trapezius.

With your hands at your sides and your thumbs pointing forward, stand with your feet about four inches apart. Press the neck together in the trunk while inhaling, then rotate the hands and shoulder blades (revolving your thumb backward) out and back again (tighten your buttocks). Exhale while you maintain this stance with your shoulders lowered.

Hold this position for approximately six seconds while inhaling and exhaling normally while moving your thoughts back to bring your hearing in line with your shoulder blades. In order to keep yourself in a relaxed state of consciousness, you should avoid shifting your nasal area or opening your mouth. Keep your body in the correct position after releasing the present. Try shifting your weight from your pumps to the balls of your feet, which will allow you to retain this stance without feeling rigid.

At least once every one to two hours, do this exercise to reinforce appropriate posture techniques throughout the day. To get the optimum results, do one repetition six or more times a day rather than six in a row.

Many health issues, such as headaches and stiff necks, can be traced back to disorders in the trapezius muscle. The trapezius muscle is a key player in the production process. While carrying weight, the glenohumeral joint girdle is held up by the upper fibers, which help prevent lowering of the girdle.

The trapezius muscles of the upper and lower trapezius form trigger points. Most of us have access to these trigger points, which are often active and position-related.

In addition to a wide range of common ailments such as chronic neck aches, stress, and cluster headaches, as well as cervical backbone pain and whiplash, these trigger variables are related to a wide range of other conditions.

Trigger points in the upper trapezius aren't difficult to find, and there's a lot you can do at home to relieve these "knots" and improve neck and shoulder mobility.

Self-Treatment for Trigger Points

This method focuses on finding the source of the pain. It is possible that a well-known pain map could be activated if this is compressed (ideally reproducing your symptoms).

Pressure is applied in a direct and sustained manner using this method.

Procedures

- Decide on the sensitive areas where you want to focus your time and efforts.

- Set up a place where the sponsor's muscles may relax and fully stretch out to their full extent.

- Until you encounter resistance, gently and steadily apply pressure to the soft point. Soreness, rather than pain, will be the sensation you get as a result of this.

- Constantly push on the sensitive point until you feel it soften and produce. This could take anywhere from a few seconds to several hours.

- When the soft/trigger point has fully yielded, repeat Steps 3–4 to increase the strain on it.

- You can improve your results by experimenting with different ways to apply pressure during these repetitions. Always proceed with caution and common sense!

In order to fully understand the nature of your trigger point discomfort, you must consider it in relation to the rest of your body. It is important to note that the methods described on this page should not be considered a substitute for professional therapy.

Trigger points can cause pain and discomfort, but there may be an underlying condition.

The best course of action is to always have a medical professional properly diagnose you. Use a buddy or a friend if you can; go to the process notes for more information (above).

Individualized Care Using Only the Fingertips

Using your fingertips (fingertips) is an excellent way to determine if you can actually feel the activation point itself, rather than just the surrounding area. There are a variety of pressure instruments available for purchase.

They're affordable and make it simple to visit a potential neighborhood. In our opinion, everyone should have a pressure tool in their arsenal!

When done in conjunction with self-treatment, stretching may assist in speeding up the healing process even if it doesn't do much to eliminate the trigger points on its own.

Always begin slowly and with extreme caution. Don't continue if you are in too much discomfort. Consider consulting a doctor if you've already been diagnosed with a debilitating ailment.

Taking charge of one's own health care

Self-management of treatment has been repeatedly proved to be important and valuable in studies. You might be surprised at how often basic strategies like those described above can be used to successfully treat an issue.

If you suffer from chronic or long-term pain, you should always seek the help of a trained specialist.

Most therapists can help you produce a self-managed treatment program and could have the ability to educate you on how to use pressure tools.

Anatomy of the Trapezius Muscle

There is a substantial problem with the trapezius muscle on both sides of the spine. When it comes to the human body, it's considered a large muscle that runs from the skull's upper occipital bone down to the lower thoracic vertebrae. It is the trapezius muscle that is responsible for spinning, securing, and moving the blade of the knife (scapula).

Triangular muscular fiber rings in the trapezius musculature exhibit distinct structural and functional characteristics. They all work together as a team. Glenohumeral joint blade and backbone motion are helped by these joints.

High-quality fibers located on the neck's posterior and lateral margins function to lift the blade, allowing us to do actions similar to a shrug.

The acromion procedure for the scapula involves the insertion of middle fibers along the superior thoracic vertebrae. To bring the glenohumeral joint closer to the spine, the center fibers retract and adduct the blade.

Fibers in the lower part of the trunk are called "inferior fibers" because they originate on lower vertebrae and travel into the spine of the scapula. By bringing the shoulder blade closer to the weak thoracic vertebrae, the inferior fibers try to depress it.

Trapezius Muscle Pain can be caused by what?

- **Pulled muscles:** Muscles can be pulled if they've been moved too far and too quickly, resulting in an injury. Severing muscle connections results in pain and a restricted range of motion; these are the most likely outcomes of severing muscle connections.

- **Stress:** When a person's muscles get nervous or tightened as a result of fear, it's a sign that they're experiencing stress. Soreness and pain in the muscles are the results of more muscular contractions. These symptoms may be exacerbated by stress, both mental and physical, which is common during times of high stress.

- Trapezius muscle pain can come from **poor posture**, as well as a host of other issues with the vertebral column and supporting muscles. Leaving a bad scenario in place for too long can lead to a permanent problem.

- **Strain**: Trapezius pain can be caused by overstretching the muscle or being too restricted. Heavy backpacks, handbags, or even a lack of bra straps might cause this.

- **Holding postures:** Muscle soreness in the trapezius can be caused by holding unnatural standing or sitting positions. Repetitive stress injury may also be referred to as this.

- In the event of a **traumatic injury**, such as a whiplash or a direct blow to the head, the trapezius muscles may be affected. As your brain is jerked back and forth, the trapezius muscle tenses up.

Identifying A Strain in The Trapezius Muscle

You'll be questioned extensively by your doctor about your discomfort, including where you feel it, why it's getting worse and why it's getting better, if you're seeking treatment for an undetected trapezius strain. As a result, doctors have a better sense of where the discomfort is coming from. In addition, a brief medical history and current prescription list can be helpful in identifying the source of the problem.

You should tell your doctor whether you play any sports or do any work that could have caused your trapezius muscle discomfort symptoms. An injury is the most common cause of a strain.

A physical examination would follow. It is important for your doctor to search for any signs of bruising in this area, and he or she will ask you how you feel when you move your hands and shoulder blades to determine how the trapezius muscle pain is generated. The ability to detect a gentle touch or a pinprick will be tested, as will other aspects of cranial neural function. In addition to extending reflexes, the muscle can also be used for power testing.

Specific tests like an MRI are not necessary if the developing neck and shoulder discomfort is not accompanied by additional indications or symptoms of the underlying illness.

Treatment of Trapezius Muscle Pain

- **Relax:** The healing process can be hampered if you put too much stress on your muscles.

Musculoskeletal pain can intensify if you don't make an attempt to relax.

- **Ice:** A simple method of relieving pain and inflammation is to simply put ice on the affected area. If you don't have a glacier pack, a towel filled with ice, or a bag of frozen veggies can suffice. A 15-to 20-minute snow treatment every two to four hours is highly advised for the part of the body in question.

- **Heat Therapy:** Muscle tension can be relieved with the use of a heated shower or towel. If you are very sensitive to temperature changes, this may extend to putting on warm clothing when it is cold. Healing and pain can both be sped up by the application of heat. You can also use temperature packs, which you can buy ready-made or make yourself by filling a small sock or bag with rice and microwaving it for only two minutes.

- **Epsom Salt:** Epsom salt, a common ingredient in warm baths, can also help relieve muscle aches and pains. The reason for this is because of its high magnesium level, which helps to alleviate aches and pains in the rest of the body's muscles. In order to get the best benefits, use Epsom salts in your shower for at least thirty minutes and soak the injured joint or body part. Achy muscles should be taken up to three times a week until the aching muscles have healed.

- **Activity Customization:** Getting enough rest and limiting the amount of time spent doing intense activities can also help. Taking regular breaks from sitting and learning how to sit with your back straight while at your table can help alleviate symptoms. You should be able to put your hands into the space at the lowest part of your body while sitting or standing erect.

- **Pain Medication:** When it comes to alleviating pain and inflammation, non-steroidal anti-inflammatory medications (NSAIDs) can be an excellent supplement. Ibuprofen (Motrin, Advil), naproxen (Aleve), and a slew of other prescription-only NSAIDs are examples of traditional NSAIDs. Working with these medicines requires that you follow your doctor's advice, and that there could be side effects.

Massage to Alleviate Trapezius Muscle Pain

The formation of uncomfortable knots or trigger points in the trapezius muscle will almost certainly lead to discomfort and agony, but this can be readily addressed with the application of pressure through massage. Never apply too much pressure while massaging; instead, use a clear vision. A good place to start is with shoulder blades, guitar neck, and thoracic spinal area exercises. Here are a few therapeutic massage methods you can try right now:

- **Golf ball:** Roll a golf ball back and forth between your trapezius muscles and a soft surface, such as the ground. To get the most benefit from this type of massage, pay attention to the area of discomfort.

- The trapezius muscle can be relaxed simply by laying down and allowing it to do the work for you. Maintain a cushion behind your head to support your throat and keep it aligned with your backbone while you speak. Touch the tender spot with your fingertips by reaching back with your hands.

- Many therapeutic massage equipment and techniques are available to assist you in reaching difficult-to-reach places, such as the trunk.

Trapezius muscle pain therapeutic massage can be done using either an electric or manual method, depending on your preference.

Exercises for Trapezius Muscle Strain

Stretching and exercising the trapezius, like other thoracic muscles, can help alleviate discomfort and stress. Trapezius muscle soreness can be alleviated with the following exercises:

- One of the best activities for relieving pain in the trapezius muscle is the glenohumeral joint shrug, which is performed by raising your shoulder blades toward your ear, tightening, and then releasing. Adding dumbbells to each hand might also help to increase the stretch.

- Standing with your feet shoulder-width apart, place a set of dumbbells on your thighs and hold them there as you perform an upright row. Dumbbells should now be raised to glenohumeral joint level in front of you, and then gently lowered again.

- While standing with your feet shoulder width apart and with your back straight, begin to move your shoulder blades up and forward in a circular motion. As a general rule, rotation should be carried out slowly and methodically. This exercise can even be done backwards.

- **Yoga neck stretches:** While seated, keep your feet apart and your arms at your sides, expand your right equip, and softly press your mind to the left until you feel an extension in your neck. Now, do the same thing on the other side. Place your hands on the trunk of your mind and gradually push forward, feeling an expansion in the throat and down the chest. Each extension should be held for around 20 to 30 seconds before being released.

Chapter 12

Scalene

As the name suggests, the scalene has three pairs of muscles in the lateral pharynx. The scalene anterior, scalene medius, and scalene posterior muscles. Scalenus minimus, a fourth muscle, can be found behind the lower portion of scalenus anterior. This muscle is sometimes overlooked. Anteriorly, the brachial plexus and subclavian artery join the subclavian vein and phrenic neuron as the muscle crosses over your first rib; this completes between your anterior and middle scalene.

Insertion

For all three Scalenus muscle divisions, the ascending cervical artery of the thyro-cervical trunk is the insertion point.

Action

In this action, the neck is flexed and rotated.

Function

Prior and middle scalene muscles contract flexibly and laterally to the same side, lifting the first rib. They also help to flex the neck. The work of the posterior scalene is to expand the next bone and tilt the neck to the same side. In addition, the sternocleidomastoid and sternocleidomastoid muscles provide an additional set of inspiratory muscles.

Pathologies

Scalene myofascial pain symptoms are a regional pain symptom wherein pain originates within the throat area and extends directly down. This issue may be a primary or secondary manifestation of cervical disease. Induced point activity in the scalene muscle group performs a large job in many chest muscle pain concerns. This muscle group and its trigger points must be thoroughly studied by a therapist before they can give their clients sound advice on issues such as back pain, glenohumeral pain, radiating equip pain, thoracic outlet symptoms, wrist pain, and hand pain.

Many clients worry that they are having cardiac symptoms as a result of these trigger factors causing pain in the upper body and difficulty breathing in and out. Possible medical conditions that could be caused by muscle pain are:

- Thoracic outlet syndrome

- Subacromial tendinitis

- Bicipital tenosynovitis

- Lateral epicondylitis

- Spasmodic thoracic kyphosis (Wryneck symptoms).

- Diabetic neuropathy in the wrist

- Cervical rib syndrome (costoclavicular symptoms)

Activities that might lead to scalene discomfort and symptoms are:

- Whiplash injuries are among the

- Coughing excessively

- Death by suffocation (people with asthma, emphysema, bronchitis, or pneumonia are especially vulnerable to problematic scalene muscles).

- When dragging or raising, keep your hands level with your waist.

- "Word-processor headaches" are caused by working for lengthy periods of time while only paying attention to one part of the brain.

- With your attention centered on one side, you may sleep comfortably on your stomach.

- Having to lug along a large bag or backpack.

- Wearing a collar or link that is appropriate.

Test for Scalene

- **Individual Position:** People are often supine, with their heads lifted and turned to the opposite side of their bodies, and their hands elevated above their heads.

- **Specialist Position:** The specialist is leaning forward and resting his or her fingertips against the client's brow.

- **Muscle Test Explanation:** The average person is asked to flex their upper body against the practitioner's light resistance.

Treatment

To get rid of your scalene, the first thing you need to do is wash your face. The goal of eliminating trigger points is to eliminate the underlying causes of the problem.

Place the tips of your fingers on the other side of your neck with your right hand. Maintain a small amount of pressure on a part of the throat that is not visible to the naked eye. Repeat on the opposite side and in a different part of the throat. Please repeat the procedure on both sides of the throat 5 to 10 times.

Before doing this stretch, it's a good idea to warm up the throat using a hot pack or heating pad for 10 to 30 minutes. It is important to practice adequate diaphragmatic breathing between stretches in order to relax the throat. To lower and anchor the make, place the hands of the stretched side under your buttocks. Put your other hand over your head so that your fingertips are speaking directly to your inner ear.

In order to extend your neck, gently pull your top and neck to the opposite side of the medial side that you wish to stretch, and relax your neck muscles as necessary to do so. Draw your ear all the way to your shoulder and listen intently.

A scalene will be targeted based on the amount of rotation your mind experiences. Change the person's direction toward the pulling apparatus to concentrate on the posterior scalene.

Shift your gaze away from the pulling handle to concentrate on the anterior scalene. Look directly at the roof or just slightly toward the pulling arm to hit the middle scalene.

When you move your head to focus on a specific muscle, see if you can find the one that feels the tightest. For a total of six to seven seconds, keep your arms extended.

Scalene takes a seat in a plush chair to get control. Your right hand should rest on the right side of your brain. During the activity, this hand acts as a stabilizer. Keeping the resistance generated by your right hands, begin to move your correct hearing toward your right glenohumeral joint. Repeat the process 8 to 12 times for each feature. Scalene muscle fitness improves your ability to support your cervical backbone, reducing the risk of a recurrence of an injury.

Another way to develop your scalene muscles is to sit or work while listening to a resistance music group. Keep the ends of the band firmly to one side to ensure that the band is unquestionably under pressure. Maintaining a natural stance of your thoughts, resist the movement of the music group. Keep this pose, relax, and replicate.

Free Bonus

Download my **"Keto Cookbook with 60+ Keto Recipes For Your Personal Enjoyment"** Ebook For **FREE!**

The **Keto Diet Cookbook** is a collection of **60+ delicious recipes** that are easy and fun to make in the comfort of your own home. It gives you the exact *recipes that you can use to prepare meals for any moment of the day, breakfast, lunch, dinner, and even dessert.*

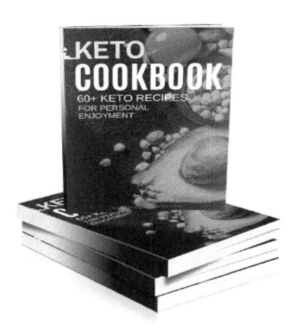

You don't need 5 different cookbooks with a ton of recipes to live a healthy and fun lifestyle. *You just need a good and efficient one and that is what the **Keto Diet***

Cookbook is.

Click the URL below to Download the Book For FREE, and also Subscribe for Free books, giveaways, and new releases by me. https://mayobook.com/drmichelle

Feedback

I'd like to express my gratitude to you for choosing to read this book, Thank you. I hope you got what you wanted from it. Your feedback as to whether I succeeded or not is greatly appreciated, as I went to great lengths to make it as helpful as possible.

<u>I would be grateful if you could write me a review on the product detail page about how this book has helped you. Your review means a lot to me, as I would love to hear about your successes.</u> Nothing makes me happier than knowing that my work has aided someone in achieving their goals and progressing in life; which would likewise motivate me to improve and serve you better, and also encourage other readers to get influenced positively by my work. <u>Your feedback means so much to me, and I will never take it for granted.</u>

However, if there is something you would love to tell me as to improve on my work, it is possible that you are not impressed enough, or you have a suggestion, errors, recommendation, or criticism for us to improve on; we are profoundly sorry for your experience (remember, we are human, we are not perfect, and we are constantly striving to improve).

Rather than leaving your displeasure feedback on the retail product page of this book, please send your feedback, suggestion, or complaint to us via E-mail to **"michelle@mayobook.com"** so that action can be taken quickly to ensure necessary correction, improvement, and implementation for the better reading experience.

I'm honored that you've read this book and that you enjoy it. I strive to provide you with the best reading experience possible.

Thank you, have a wonderful day!

About The Author

I help people to eat healthy food and live healthier lives. I have been a registered dietitian since 2005. In the past decade, I have helped hundreds of people to improve their health and wellbeing through nutrition. I am a licensed dietitian in the state of California and a member of the American Dietetic Association. I have been working in the wellness industry for over 10 years, and I have worked with people who have type 2 diabetes, high blood pressure, heart disease, weight gain, metabolic syndrome, and cancer. I understand that nutrition is key to good health, and I love helping people eat well.

My goal is to help people get healthy by providing them with a balanced diet, lifestyle changes, and support. My approach is holistic, which means that I look at diet as a whole, rather than focusing on one aspect.

I am a holistic nutritionist. I help people change their eating habits and lifestyles so they can achieve and maintain a healthy weight and a happy, energetic lifestyle. I teach people how to eat well, and I help people find the balance between healthy food and food that they love. I also work with people who have cancer, diabetes, and other chronic conditions to help them live healthier lives. I offer personalized nutrition counseling and healthy meal planning. I have a master's degree in nutrition and a doctorate in nutritional science. I am a registered dietitian in the state of California and a member of the American Dietetic Association. I believe in a healthy lifestyle, and I help people find the best path to get there.

Subscribe to my Newsletter to download my Free Book, and also be informed about my new releases, and giveaways here: https://mayobook.com/drmichelle

Connect with me on my Facebook Page here: https://fb.me/MichelleEllenGleen

My Books

Alkaline Diet: The Secret to Healthy Living with Alkaline Foods (Healthy Food Lifestyle)

The Alkaline Diet Cookbook: Your Guide to Eating More Alkaline Foods, and Less Acidic Foods For Healthy Living (Healthy Food Lifestyle)

Ketogenic Diet For Beginners: Your Complete Keto Guide and Cookbook with Low Carb, High-Fat Recipes For Living The Keto Lifestyle

Anti Inflammatory Diet Cookbook For Beginners: 3-Week Quick & Delicious Meal Plan with Easy Recipes to Heal The Immune Systems and Restore Overall Health

Apple Cider Vinegar: A Quick, Easy, and Affordable Guide to the Health Benefits, and Healing Power of Apple Cider Vinegar (ACV)

Apple Cider Vinegar: The Amazing Guide on The Uses of ACV For Numerous Health Conditions, and How to Make it from Home

Brain Cancer Awareness: How to Help Your Brain Fight Brain Cancer

Dr. Sebi Cookbook: Alkaline Diet Nutritional Guide with Sea moss, Medicinal Herbal Teas, Smoothies, Desserts, Mushroom, Salads, Soups & More, to Rejuvenate the Body with 100+ Recipes

Skin Tag Removal: How To Get Rid of Your Skin Tags in Simple

Steps

Trigger Points: The New Self Treatment Guide to Pain Relief

CPSIA information can be obtained
at www.ICGtesting.com
Printed in the USA
LVHW080852230123
737741LV00008B/361

9 781637 503447